GOOD HAIR

GOOD HAIR

FOR COLORED GIRLS
WHO'VE CONSIDERED WEAVES
WHEN THE CHEMICALS
BECAME TOO RUFF

Lonnice Brittenum Bonner

THREE RIVERS PRESS

NEW YORK

Published by Three Rivers Press, New York, New York.
Member of the Crown Publishing Group.

Random House, Inc. New York, Toronto, London, Sydney, Auckland
www.randomhouse.com

THREE RIVERS PRESS is a registered trademark and the Three Rivers Press colophon is a trademark of Random House, Inc.

Originally published by Sapphire Publications in 1992.

Printed in the United States of America.

Library of Congress Cataloging-in-Publication Data
Bonner, Lonnice Brittenum.
Good hair: for colored girls who've considered weaves when the chemicals became too ruff / by Lonnice Brittenum Bonner.
Reprint. Originally published: Oakland, CA: Sapphire Publications, © 1991.
Includes bibliographical references.
1. Hairdressing of African-Americans. I. Title.
TT972.B65   1994   646.7'24'08996073—dc20   93-42027

ISBN 0-517-88151-9

15 14 13 12

ACKNOWLEDGMENTS

The author wishes to thank the following people for their support.

My parents, Lonnie and Dorothy Brittenum
my brother, Demoine C. Brittenum

Martha R. Blanding
Mary R. Blanding
Robert O. Blanding
Fred and Nellie Bonner
Capril Bonner-Thomas
Angel Braestrup
Lawrence Braxton
Milicent Chamble
Edward and Bernice Daniels
Gerald and Patricia Davis
Luella Davis
William Drummond and Faith Fancher
Tammerlin Drummond
Mary Mach
Doris G. Worsham
Thelma Simmons
Peggy Dillard Toone
DeKar Lawson, Lee Priestly, Jennifer Ashby

PHOTO CREDITS: Victor Hall, Auintard Henderson
COVER GRAPHICS: Cassandra Chavez
COVER DESIGN: Lonnice Brittenum Bonner
LAYOUT: Canterbury Press, Berkeley, California

FOR
MY PARENTS

and

DEREK
who would not
let me quit

TABLE OF CONTENTS

GOOD HAIR

INTRODUCTION

For Colored Girls
Who've Considered Weaves
When The Chemicals Became Too Ruff

Every Black woman wants good hair. We already have it, but most of us claim it is too much trouble to care for unless the texture is radically or chemically altered. Many women would prefer to have chronically damaged, unflattering hair, styled in what they believe is an "acceptable" manner. This is unfortunate.

What does "good hair" mean? It means hair that is the best it can be, hair that's healthy looking, a natural adornment.

Notice that I **didn't** refer to hair of a certain texture or "grade" as if our hair should be graded like a piece of USDA choice meat. If you can manage and enjoy your hair without going though major changes, then I'd say it's pretty good.

I used to think only Black women with so-called "good hair" were the luckiest women in the world. You know what I mean. Hair that's naturally straight, loosely curled or waved. Those of us with the springy African hair were banished to "bad hair" purgatory, doomed to spend eternity trying to make it look "good." Then, there's the faction that has deemed anything less than straight hair, to be "political" hair. Let me translate: political equals **militant** and we don't want to offend the wrong people, do we? Men don't like women whose hair looks like **that!**

For those of us blessed with African hair, this program can really get on your nerves. Hey, I just want to look good. Why does looking good mean I've gotta look like someone else? All rationalizing aside, isn't imitation the sincerest form of flattery? You'd think that the last thing we'd want to do is spend lots of time and hard earned cash doing bad hair imitations. I mean, what's a sista ta do?

First off, knowledge is power and what you don't know about your own hair can hurt you, or at least your pocketbook. Consider this: Black hair care is a billion dollar business. Also consider the fact that white people are very aware of our desire for so called "good hair." Because Blacks tend to spend more on hair care than whites, white owned companies have already begun to target the Black hair care market, which now grosses more than $1 billion a year and there are no signs of decline.

But even though Black women spend a lot of money on hair care it seems that money can't buy miracles. So many ladies have ruined their hair with improperly applied chemical straighteners, curly perms and dyes that someone figured they'd buy glue-on bangs if made available.

We're not talking about Black women with medical or dermatological problems that affect hair growth. We're talking about healthy, intelligent women who believe that there is basically one way to wear their hair — straightened —and are overwhelmed by all the chemical services that purportedly work miracles and have a hard time finding professionals who take time to do the job right.

Just try counting the ads for hair growth aids or quick fix weaves and wigs in any magazine or media oriented toward Black women. How many ladies do you know who've suddenly switched hairdressers midstream because someone whispered those magic words —"Girlfriend, my hair has really **grown** since I've been going to Tyrell. And he gets you out **quick!**"

But for all the time and considerable cash we spend on our hair, you can see millions of sisters with, well, let us say serious hair problems. Let me give you a few highlights from my own experiences:

▶ When I let a hair stylist convince me that cutting one side of my hair radically shorter than the other would make it grow in faster and thicker than the uncut side. I am ashamed to say I was a working journalist at the time, because "bogus" was written all over this one. And no, it didn't work.

▶ When I wore braids for one and a half years and grew a shoulder-length head of hair I literally thanked God for, only to screw it right up with a chemical straightener ... on top of a home curly perm. Go ahead and snicker, but you know women who've done this if you haven't already done it yourself...

▶ The times I've gone to work with big, dark burn marks on my forehead and neck, where my curling iron slipped. If my hair had been long enough to hide my forehead and neck, it would have been bearable. The shame of this was that I got the ultra short relaxed style so I wouldn't have to fool with curling irons and rollers in the first place.

▶ How about the time I went into a salon for a mild relaxer and wedge cut and came out with the tightest, greasiest curly perm — I can't bear to go on, it was so awful. My hair just kind of sat up on the back of my head like it was disgusted. My husband, a very tolerant man, refused to touch it. My hair was so parched, it drank quarts of curl activator. I couldn't wait until I got a couple inches of growth so I could cut the greasy mess off. Another complete head of hair bit the dust.

But the killer, the absolute clincher was when I thumbed through one of those "true love" confessional magazines aimed at Black women and found an ad for —my hand to God—glue on hair tendrils. For about $24, you could send in for **strands**, mere tendrils of hair, to glue on at your temples and nape of your neck. That's right, for you sisters who've literally burned out your hairline behind chemical straighteners or face lifting braid extensions, there's hope! Hallelujah! According to the ad, which ran, not in 1959 but 1989, you could put a bunch of these tendrils together and glue on some bangs. This is a sorry state of affairs and I knew there must be a lot of ladies looking for help.

So this book is about learning to get control of your hair and feel good about it, enjoy it. You can be confident that if you have it cut into a style, you can enjoy it and when it grows out you can try another cut. You don't have to plan your lifestyle around your hair style but you do need a plan. That's where this book comes in. Your goal is to either:

1. Learn to manage your own hair or...

2. Educate yourself so you can't be finessed or faked out at the salon or...

3. Get "bad hair" out of your vocabulary.

4. Get off the perm and into unstraightened, or at the most, slightly texturized African hair.

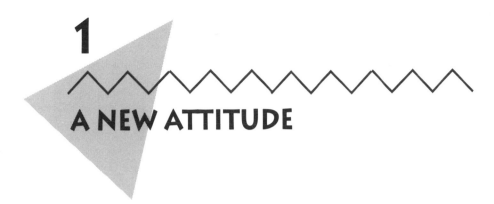

1

A NEW ATTITUDE

The key to enjoying your hair is a positive attitude. For some of you, this means a **new** attitude. Yes, ladies, there is an attitude amongst us and it manifests itself in the way of a notorious disease. It's called "Nappy Hair Phobia," also known as "Fear of Naps." I'll call it NHP for short. What causes NHP? Is there a cure?

Let's get to the root of the problem. NHP usually starts in early childhood. Mothers bearing the instrument of torture — an Ace comb — closed in on unsuspecting toddlers with curly African hair. Once caught, the poor babies were subjected to their first genuine hair combing. Toddlers blessed with strong, springy hair were in double jeopardy. Not only did they have "really bad hair" but if they cried, their mothers declared they were "tender headed." Your head would feel tender too if you tried to pull **your** springs through an Ace comb! Thus, begins the no-win game of Hair Stratego — Keisha sees Mommy coming with the Ace comb, Keisha runs away and cries. The squirming and crying gets on Mommy's nerves, so she grooms less frequently and Keisha's hair goes it's own way. Keisha sees Mommy coming with the comb... Of course nowadays, when Keisha starts the squirming and crying, Moms gets Keisha some heavy duty braid extensions — 'cause Keisha doesn't have enough hair for her own braids — or worse, a scary curl.

Then comes childhood. Who can forget the words that have terrorized generations of Black children: "Sit down so I can comb your hair." Those with curly African hair were usually treated to a half hour of having their head jerked and snatched, while Mother struggled through the crop. Moms would be talking 'bout how "you must have gotten your **father's** hair—they've got that **bad** hair" or "this stuff is so nappy I can hardly get the comb through it!" Pow! "Hold your head up straight!"

I understand where the attitude comes from because I have been there too. Hair outlaws are created, not born.

I am a child of the integration era who went to school with white kids. I lived in predominately white neighborhoods. I was getting my hair pressed back then, so I got the "good hair" culture shock first hand — I quickly discovered that my hair didn't do what it was "supposed" to do — stay straight.

Hair care was very important because naps were not in vogue. You did not want your white classmates asking you why your hair looked like **that.** My mother took great pains to be sure our secret wasn't revealed. When I started school, she made a black drawstring bag and slipped a folded raincoat inside. I carried this bag to school **every day**, rain or shine. Heaven forbid if it should drizzle and my hair were to go back. I'd have go back to wherever it came from.

My mother has thick, pretty black hair that she —get this— prefers to wear short because she says it's "too much trouble" when it's long. Every once in a while, she'd let it grow past her shoulders and then she'd whack it off short. This drove me crazy. The luck of the gene pool gave me my grandmamma's fragile hair. It's what folks call "soft" hair. To me, it was about as good as having soft teeth. Give it a hard press, a good oiling and it would cling to my skull like white on rice. My nickname was "Go 'head, fo'head" because I have —ahem—what is known as an intelligent forehead. And once I began doing my own hair, I didn't have much fringe to cover it.

Ah, the hot comb. I remember it well. My mom would give me the 'do that most Black girl children get —the two or three plaits and the ubiquitous rolled bang. My mom believed that more than three plaits looked like Buckwheat and y'all know that was definitely **out** back then.

I remember walking to school winter mornings and feeling the grease freeze in my bangs —excuse me, I meant my **bang.**

Speaking of bangs, there's an impression amongst us that hair can be "trained." That is, instead of cutting your bangs and having them fall into place, Black people trim their bangs and "train" them so they'll lay **right.** In my case, part of this "training" involved a device called the stocking cap.

One of my earliest training memories is of my mother making me a stocking cap to sleep in. Now, we're not talking about the knit cap that Wee Willie Winkle wore with the little pom pom on top. I'm talking about the kind made from a real stocking. My mom would take one of her stockings, cut off the leg and knot the top to create a little cap. I was what some people call a "bad sleeper," so she'd make a chin strap with a piece of elastic.

The chin strap was for my mom's peace of mind, because

I was already getting a nightly face lift from the stocking cap. The rationale behind this was to keep my hair — and the rollers or pin curls — in place while I slept. It also "trained" my bangs by immobilizing them against my forehead — **nothing** was gonna move under that little baby. That's when that bang training really came into good use — training my bangs to cover the forehead ring and roller marks pressed in by the stocking cap.

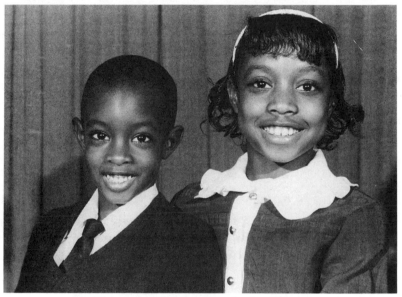

Me, my brother and my trained bangs

I eventually graduated to sleepwear designed by Goody Hair Products. Some of these fashion innovations included what they called a "sleep bonnet." This was a synthetic shower cap covered with the scratchiest, ugliest eyelet material ever invented. At least they didn't come with chin straps.

I can really relate to Whoopi Goldberg's joke about wearing a towel on her head, pretending it was her hair because I did that stuff too. Y'all probably did it unless you were born in the 70's and your mother got you some braid extensions. Well, my version of The Towel was to tie a big thick ribbon or yarn-tie on the end of my finger-length, dookie braid and flip **that** around. Except I didn't have sense enough to keep it at home, I wore mine to school... until somebody drew a picture of me with the huge yarn bow dangling on the back of my microscopic braid....

I grew up believing that grease grew hair and if I could just find the magic brand I'd be Rapunzel's twin sister. Our house brand was the standard cool blue, Ultra Sheen. Wasn't no Afro Sheen for me 'cause my mom didn't especially go for no great big nappy looking Afros. Besides, I didn't have no great big hair to Afro with anyhow. Anyway, I faithfully brushed and oiled my little crop with the Ultra Sheen until one of my girlfriends told me a grease called Sulfur 8 made her hair grow. If you don't know about Sulfur 8, the name speaks for itself. It's feels great on an itchy scalp. But once it's aged a few days in your hair, it's hard to keep Sulfur 8 a secret. And don't let it be a hot day.

Glover's Mange was another favorite hair grower. When my mom put some warmed Glover's on a cotton pad and rubbed it into my scalp it was better than having my feet rubbed — I swore new hairs were sprouting. Until I looked at my crop two weeks later and it looked the same , short-n-skimpy.

I was also a brush disciple —100 strokes a night. After my hair was hot combed, before the grease was put in, I'd run around the house, shaking my three inches of hair (that's about the longest it ever got.) I'd watch it shake and bounce like the white girls' hair. Then my mother would oil my scalp and spoil my fantasy. The Ultra Sheen would be brushed though, ("so it won't go back so fast") and then I'd roll it up on sponge rollers. I slept on sponge rollers **every** night. To prevent the sponge from chewing up my hair — very important step here — I'd fold a section of toilet paper in half and wrap it around the roller. It was the only way to ensure a hair style in the morning because I sure didn't have enough to slick into a bun if the set didn't work.

When I was a teenager, a lady I babysat for gave me a curly brown Afro wig. My mom gave me the high sign because wigs were in and many of her friends wore wigs. We're talking about the wig heyday here, starring "It's a Wig" by Michael Weeks, the Naomi Sims line and so on. With my new hair and fake fur bomber jacket, I looked just like my movie idol, Cleopatra Jones! Honey, I was **too** fine! And as an added bonus, my girlfriend told me if I kept my hair braided up underneath the wig, it would grow! I had been reborn.

Ladies, I had the time of my life. I went to a skating rink with my wig on and a G.I. tried to pick me up. I was all of 14-years-old at the time. Prior to that time (we'll call it "B.H." —before hair) I couldn't pay a brother to ask me to dance at a party. Ah, the miracle of hair!

The problem was that everybody who knew me, knew it was a wig. So I had to be extra cool — I didn't want anybody getting riled up and snatching it off to make a point. Also, any boys I pulled would want to run their hands through my bountiful hair sooner or later. And lastly, the sucker had to be washed and I didn't have an alternate to wear while it dried.

When I found out about hair weaves, that you could actually attach hair to your head and not have to take it off at night, I became obsessed. I pouted for a month one summer until my mother threatened to give me a reason to need one.

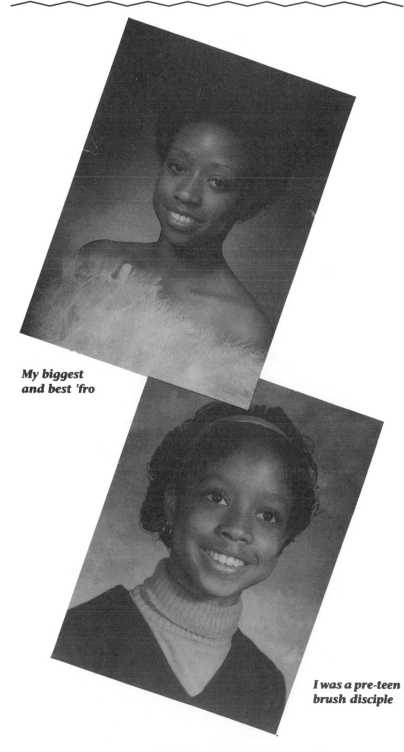

*My biggest
and best 'fro*

*I was a pre-teen
brush disciple*

I could go on, but I'll stop here while I still have some secrets left.

It's no wonder that many of us wanted to get rid of "the problem." The mission: Get those naps out and put some curls in. Unfortunately, the curls were already there — we just didn't know how to work with them and we didn't **want** to.

It's difficult to stop Black hair from breaking off when it's constantly styled with chemical straighteners and lots of heat from blow dryers and curling irons. It you hate African hair, then you're more likely to wear it out by using harsh styling methods to keep it straight.

Now when your hair is constantly breaking off from styling methods, you get the impression that it doesn't grow. Believing that your hair doesn't grow is a downer, don't you think? So then you tend to feel trapped into a hair style. It's like you don't have a choice or the **luxury** of letting your hair grow so you can try something different. If you don't see any attractiveness in your own hair, you turn to quick fixes like weaves and wigs. You figure Black women with healthy, pretty hair or straight hair, have "good hair." It couldn't possibly be better because they **treat it better**. You develop bad feelings about your hair.

NHP has a way of cropping up in ways you probably recognize. Here are a few of the dreadful styling diseases that promote the image of springy African hair as a burden to be disguised.

✂ **RELAXER REVENGE** This happens when the urge to purge the naps is so great that you overprocess your chemical relaxer to the point of no return. Symptoms are a burnt out hairline or a balding look around the sides. Victims of Relaxer Revenge often sport a 'do that is brittle and stiff or like greased cake icing.

✄ **THE NAP STRIKES BACK** The best description I've heard is when your hair has "reverted to an Uncle Remus style nap." Strikeback sufferers usually try to brush or grease the naps into what's left of their bone straight perm.

✄ **IMITATION OF STILL LIFE** Often confused with its close cousin, Relaxer Revenge, The Imitation stems from the sister's fear of naps, haircuts, trims or scissors in general. The Imitators credo: Why cut if you can **comb**? So you see faithfully bad recreations of the latest hair fad. Who can forget the Farrah Fawcett era? Feats of magic were performed as countless sisters created the immortal winged flip out of what in some cases was literally thin air. Then we had the trend where we saw three and four different hair styles on one head —bangs in front, layers on the left, blunt pageboy to the right, no back. All without benefit of scissors. Relaxer Revenge victims really lucked out during that era because they could usually count on their hair just kinda breaking off into a 'do, thus saving them the heartbreak of a trim or haircut.

✄ **STRETCH AND SAVE SYNDROME** Also known as see-through hair.

"Yeah girl, it's down to my shoulders now." But it's so broken and damaged that you can see through the last five inches of it.

✄ **THE BABY HAIR MYSTIQUE** An abundance of "baby hair" the soft downy hair that lies along the hairline and nape, is admired among us. When it occurs naturally, it is naturally attractive. But some of us get carried away. Like the pitiful sisters who don't have enough hair to catch up in a baby barrette but have worked miracles with a lotta styling gel and what's left of their hairline. And no example of the Baby Hair Mystique would be complete without mentioning Michael Jackson.

I believe NHP exists because we see so few examples of desirable hair styles that highlight the natural texture of curly African hair. Most of us have been conditioned to admire African hair after it has been completely straightened. There doesn't seem to be an easy in-between. I'm not into measuring negritude by hairstyles. I'm saying that every Black woman in America doesn't necessarily want to wear her hair like Claire Huxtable. I'm also saying that every Black woman in America with short hair doesn't want to go out, get some braid extensions, unbraid them to about one or two inches from the scalp, brush it out and curl the extensions so it looks like Claire Huxtable's.

So enough already. Before we get to the promised land, you should know something about the unique structure of African hair. Read on.

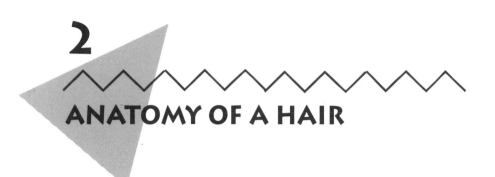

2

ANATOMY OF A HAIR

Ever wonder....

▶ Why African hair doesn't shine like naturally straight hair?

▶ Why it tends to be so dry?

▶ Why it tangles so easily, especially when it's be processed?

▶ Why processed hair breaks so easily?

▶ Why oiling your scalp is a waste of time?

These mysteries can be solved when you understand how African hair is structured. Contrary to popular belief, African hair is not the headache that those hair straightener commercials lead you to believe it is. What is unique about African hair is its *degree of curliness*. Period. Remember exponential numbers in math class? Well, African hair is hair that is curly to the *nth* degree. Welcome to Hair Anatomy 101. And remember ladies, if you know the basics, you'll save yourself a *lot* of hair. Trust me...

We'll start with the root. (see illustration) Each hair grows from a FOLLICLE, which is the pore from which the hair emerges. The root of the hair is called the PAPILLA. When you pull out a hair, the whitish bulb you see is what remains of the papilla. Each hair follicle is nourished by a SEBACEOUS GLAND that oozes an oily waxy substance called SEBUM. If your hair feels dirty and you scratch your scalp, you can see the oily sebum underneath your fingernails.

The hair shaft itself is made of KERATIN, a fibrous protein. Your fingernails and toenails are also made of keratin.

Your hair shaft is made up of three different layers of keratin. The outside layer is the CUTICLE. The cuticle contains your hair's pigment. When magnified, it looks like tiny shingles.

Anatomy of a Hair

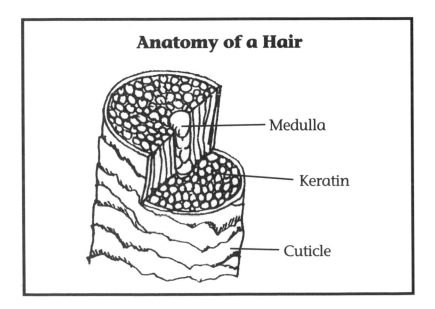

— Medulla

— Keratin

— Cuticle

The layer underneath the cuticle is called the CORTEX. The cortex is a bunch of rope like fibers that determine the thickness or thinness of your hair shaft. For example, women with fine, baby soft hair have hairs with a thinner cortex. Women with coarse or wiry hair have thicker cortexes. Many African women with fine hair think it is coarse because it is excessively curly.

The middle or core of the hair shaft is called the MEDULLA. It is a soft keratin layer.

▶ Curly, wavy or straight

The shape of the indvidual hair shafts is what determines
if your hair is curly, wavy or straight. Curly hair comes out of an almost flat shaped follicle. Straight hair comes out of a round follicle and wavy stems from an oval follicle. (see illustration)

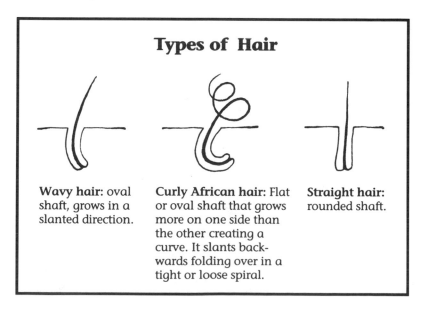

Types of Hair

Wavy hair: oval shaft, grows in a slanted direction.

Curly African hair: Flat or oval shaft that grows more on one side than the other creating a curve. It slants backwards folding over in a tight or loose spiral.

Straight hair: rounded shaft.

You can have curly hair with some naturally wavy sections or a head of straight hair with some waves. There are many degrees of curliness in African hair, ranging from wavy to very tight, watchspring coils. Kinky African hair is hair that is *excessively* curly or curly to the *nth* degree. If you pull out a strand of unprocessed African hair, it looks like a coiled spring or a Slinky toy. Because of its structure, you'll get the best results it you treat Black hair like curly hair instead of always going the extreme opposite.

Many women with tight African hair actually have two or three degrees of curl on different parts of their scalp. For instance, when I grew a head of unprocessed hair, I discovered that the curls on the crown of my head and nape of my neck were looser than on the sides and back.

▶ So, why is African hair so dry? Why is oiling the scalp a waste of time?

Sebum, the oily, waxy substance from your oil follicles, works its way down the hair shaft to lubricate the hair. If you hair is naturally straight, the sebum flows straight down, without any interruption.

But African hair is built like a coiled spring. Instead of flowing down, it must work its way around each twist and turn of the curl. Most of the time, the oil never makes it to the ends, so the hair feels dry, even when the scalp is oily. That's why oiling your scalp is a waste of time. I'll show you a smarter way to lubricate your hair and stimulate your scalp later.

Even when African hair is chemically straightened, the dryness problem isn't solved. The chemicals break down the keratin bonds in the cuticle so the curls will straighten out.

The loss of keratin and the chemical process make your hair shaft dryer because the protective shingles are altered. So even though sebum can flow down your straightened hair shaft, it isn't enough to correct the chemically induced dryness.

▶ Why doesn't African hair shine more?

Light hits the shingles on straight hair and refracts off them like light refracts off a pane of smooth glass. If your hair is excessively curly, the light must reflect off of the twist and turns and the shiny effect is diminished. But your hair will still have a healthy gleam if it's in good condition. Sometimes African-American women will glop on the oil or pomade, trying to get the same shine that women with naturally straight hair have, but it just looks greasy instead of shiny. It's better to apply a transparent color glaze or try one of the new shine products containing silicone instead.

▶ Why does African hair break so easily, especially when chemically processed? Why does it tangle so much?

When your hair is in bad condition, or has been overprocessed, the cuticle shingles won't lie down and sometimes parts of it will be missing. The opened shingles will catch onto the roughened shingles of other hairs and it will tangle easily. The inner layers of your hair are unprotected and your hair will break easily.

Chemically processed hair is *especially* delicate when wet. When water hits the already weakened bonds become like limp strings. In overprocessed or damaged hair, the wet strands are like limp, spongy spaghetti.

If your hair has not been chemically processed, the springy curls simply coil around each other, especially when your hair is dry. Each twist and turn of the spring is a weak spot. However, it's still better off breakage-wise than processed hair. If you wet your hair, the moisture helps to soften it and it is much easier to comb through and untangle.

Gee, sounds like some heavy deal, doesn't it? Don't let it overwhelm you, because as I said, the secret is to go with the flow. In other words, treat your hair the way it was meant to be treated and you'll enjoy it.

Now, you're probably thinking, "I don't want to be bothered — isn't there something *easy* I can do, something **quick?**" Remember, that's the attitude that brought you here in the first place. Let's talk about what "quick and easy" will get you....

3

IF YOU GIVE A DANCE
YOU GOTTA PAY THE BAND

One thing that really bugs ladies is getting a hairstyle they think is really cute and appears to be low maintenance, but packs a sneaky punch in time and money. For example, a curly perm seems footloose and fancy free, until you consider little necessities like curl activator, curl moisturizer, protein conditioners, the jheri curl shampoo, new pillowcases and plastic shower caps. If you can evaluate the costs and benefits going in, you can make a more satisfying choice.

You should also understand that when you choose a hair style that requires little or no chemical alteration you'll spend some time adjusting to new styling techniques. If you've been accustomed to straightened hair and depending upon hot curlers and blow dryers to create a style, you're going to fumble a bit at first. But don't give up! The tradeoff —length, versatility, style and gradually, less styling time— is worth it.

I've discovered that the only hair style for Black women that can be done with no real time investment is a quo vadis or an ultra short natural. These are tried and true "wash -

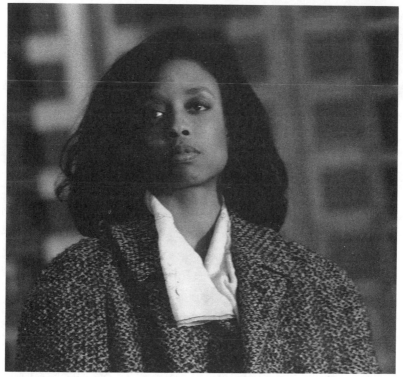

The Great Pretender
If I look grim, it's because this style demands major upkeep.

n-go" hair styles and you can eliminate those trips to the salon with a frugal purchase of hair clippers and a good friend with a steady hand. Even dreadlocks take time and care if you want them to look good. Here's my experience with one well known "wash-n-go" style, the mighty braid extensions.

When I wore braids for the first time, I thought I'd died and gone to heaven. I went to Back to Braids in Los Angeles (no longer in business) and got one layer of tiny cornrows (no scalp showing) and an off the center part. Thanks to the miracle of extensions,. I had braids past my shoulders. So what if it took almost 12 hours and $125 of my hard earned dollars—we're talkin' serious wash and go! No more shower caps! Rain and fog became my friends! Last one in the water was a rotten egg!

Now, I couldn't really brush to get the dandruff off my scalp but no-o-o problem—just put a little oil between the rows and the itching would stop. Shampooing? No problem! Hey, it's wash and *go!* Just shampoo, tie a scarf down on the braids to keep the frizzies down while it dried—then, off I'd go.

Then, the really neat stuff started happening — my hair began to grow! For the first time in my life, I could actually see a whole inch of my own hair underneath the cornrowed extensions. All this after only two months! What it really meant was that it was time to take the braids out, but heck, why screw things up when they were just starting to get good? Plus, I got a **lot** of rap action behind my braids; men loved them. They were different, they were exotic. I loved my braids — I **needed** my braids. How was I going to go back to my own short, boring hair after all this?

Three and a half months later ...

The scarf trick wasn't working anymore and it began to look like the cornrows were floating an inch above my scalp. It took **TWO DAYS** to take the braids out. My fingers cramped up pulling out masses of shedded hair and caked dandruff that couldn't be rinsed away because of the cornrows. But I was so attached to having all that hair to fling over my shoulder that I vowed I would go through it all again. I wore braids for a year and a half.

In retrospect, the pleasure I received from the braids outweighed the upkeep and my hair did get a rest from harsh chemical straighteners. But I did pay for "convenience."

One price was no versatility. Once I had braids, I was

stuck with the style until it was time to take them out.

Another price was my time. Sure, daily grooming was a snap. But it all caught up with me when it was time to take them out. It took at least a day, that night and the better part of the next day to take them down properly. This included washing and conditioning, all done by yours truly. It's is very expensive to have a professional take braids out for you. Most will charge about $25 an hour and if you've ever taken out small braids it seems like it takes an hour just to take **one** braid out.

Yet another price was being totally dependent upon someone else to get my hair done. You can be sure nobody saw me or my head from the time I took the braids out until the time I got them redone. If I didn't want to answer questions about my suddenly short hair, I had to carefully plan and scheme two or three consecutive days off to take the suckers out, wash and condition, trim and re-braid. And it was at **their** convenience, not mine. If you've ever had your hair braided outside a salon, you know that the braider doesn't start braiding when you sit down and continue until the style is done. Somehow, phones, children, trips to the store and everything else interferes. A braider also tends to stop when **she** gets tired, even if she hasn't finished your hair. That means you have to go home and come back the next day.

Like it or not, all hair styles are going to require time, even the styles that seem quick and easy. If you have turned to this book for inspiration in finding another alternative, you know that trying for quick and easy will take you back to where you started from — trying to find a style, any style to hide damage or giving up and wearing the old blowdry and curling iron 'do.

Look at it this way, if you take time to care for you hair

it shows in a big way. And if you notice women who have pretty, sexy hair, it **looks** natural; it doesn't scream "processed!" even if it is. But they still spend time with it. One woman may say, "I don't blow dry it — it doesn't take time at all." That means she takes time to let it dry naturally because she knows that blow drying is harsh and will dry out her hair.

Ask yourself a few questions *before* you consider a less chemically dependent hair style.

▶ Do you hate spending any time with your hair? If you don't like to do your hair at all, you'd be better off with a short natural or some of the jazzy new short natural cuts that require a trip to the barber or 30 minutes in a salon chair.

▶ Are you known as Miss Trendsetter? Braids this month, marcelled waves next, then a poker-straight bob? Then you need versatility, and you can't lock yourself into a serious chemical jones by doing irreversible stuff like curly perms.

▶ Do you dream of long hair? If you do, you're going to have to make a commitment of *at least* 18 months. Period. That means taking time to de-tangle with your fingers, taking time to protect the ends, avoiding styling methods that require heat.

I've had a lot of stuff done to my hair — weaves, braids, curly perms, relaxers, press and curls, natural and even TWA — teeny weeny Afro. The time I spend on my hair now is nothing compared to the headaches and disappointments I got from going "quick and easy."

4

TOOLS OF THE TRADE

The gentlest, safest tools you can use on your hair are your own hands. If you are interested in hair that grows instead of breaks, you will quickly learn how to section and detangle your hair with your fingers.

In my experience there are a few things you should have for daily hair maintenance. A good rule of thumb is to think **gentle** when choosing hair tools, things that won't catch onto curly hair, materials that are smooth, plastics that have no rough edges. Remember, most problems with African hair stem from subtle, gradual, daily abuse. Beauty supply stores usually have the best selection of tools to choose from as well as a pretty good price range. Here's my list:

THE HAIR TOOL BOX

A PLASTIC, WIDE-TOOTHED COMB — make sure it's of good quality by examining between the teeth for sharp plastic edges. Run the comb over the back of your hand to see if it scratches. If the teeth are needle sharp, you can only imagine what they will do to your scalp and hair.

A GENTLE, NATURAL BRISTLE BRUSH — I had always heard that you should use a natural bristle brush every day, so you can distribute scalp oils throughout your hair. I was a faithful disciple of this edict for many years and for years there was more hair in my brush than on my head. Then I visited a dear aunt and uncle in Tennessee and noticed that my uncle used a baby hair brush. I didn't notice much hair in his brush, so I got one. My version is a natural bristle complexion brush. I reasoned that bristles that are gentle to the complexion would be easy on the scalp and hair. I realize that some of you may be blessed with stronger hair than mine and may be able to use a stiffer brush and keep your hair. Use whatever works for you.

BEDTIME HAIR CARE — Girlfriends, I know you want to get away from wearing a "rag" on your head in bed. But he can't run his fingers through it noways if you don't have anything for him to run them through! Here's what you do; put your scarf under the pillow and put it on after he's done running his fingers through your locks or at least get a proper pillowcase. Read on.

PILLOWCASES: When your hair lays unprotected on a cotton pillowcase, the hair catches onto the tiny cotton fibers and breaks. It is doubly abusive to chemically straightened hair. What we're talking about here is **gradual** damage. The absorbent cotton material also absorbs any protective oils your scalp may secrete. In short, it helps the breakage cycle along.

BETTER CHOICE: Get a satin pillowcase. As you know, satin and silk are the gentlest materials when it comes to your hair. You may also find that a satin pillow cover will help curls and waves stay intact because the satin weave allows your hair to **slide over** the fabric. And it doesn't have to cost a fortune — you can pick up a satin pillow cover for about five to ten dollars at most department stores. If you are rich, you can spring for actual pillowcases and matching sheets.

SCARVES: Start collecting great looking scarves to wear and sleep in. Pick them up at second hand stores for anywhere from fifty cents to three dollars. If you have a satin pillow cover you can get away from wearing a scarf most of the time. However, if your hair is in that in-between length and too short to put up for sleeping, you may find that wearing a scarf helps your curls and waves last longer.

HAIRPINS — Avoid using metal bobby pins and hair pins. The only kind I will use in a pinch are the metal kind with two crimped prongs, not the kind with a crimped prong and a flat prong. Some hair care experts say you can use the latter type as long as the plastic tips remain on the ends, but

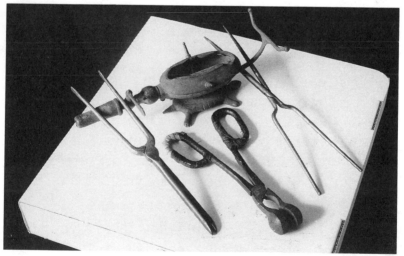

Tools of Antiquity.
Antique gas jet heater with curling irons and "pullers." Before the hot comb, your hair was pullled through this mean looking tool in order to straighten it.

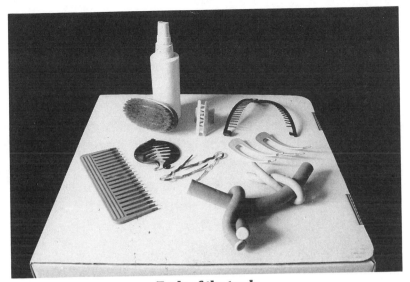

Tools of the trade.
Clockwise, lower left: comb, faux tortoiseshell hairpins and hairclip,
gentle hairbrush, squirt bottle, plastic "clippie", plastic hairpins and
flexible rubber rollers.

I find this to be a waste of time and hair. The edges of the flattened metal hair pins rub against your hair shafts like little knives and break them off.

BETTER CHOICE: Use the faux plastic tortoiseshell hair pins. You can find them at the barrette display in beauty supply stores, department stores and better drug stores. The smallest ones are a bit larger than metal bobby pins and they also come in sizes large enough to anchor an upsweep. They cost about three to four dollars a pair, but they will last much longer than the metal variety, you won't lose them as easily and they'll keep hair on your head.

SPRITZ WATER BOTTLE — Use the water spritz when you want to dampen all or part of your hair for de-tangling or re-styling. The key to faster drying is not to saturate your hair but to <u>mist</u> it. You can buy spritz bottles from the beauty supply or drug store or you can recycle one from an old pump hair spray bottle. Remember, you want a spray head that <u>mists</u>, so choose accordingly. Some spritz bottles have adjustable spray heads.

A DETACHABLE SHOWER HEAD — Whether you plan to maintain your hair between visits to a professional or enjoy doing it yourself, buying a detachable shower head is one of the best investments you can make. It's a real pain to pirouette under a fixed shower head with soap in your eyes, hoping the water is hitting the right spots. Get the type that adjusts to a pulsating water flow. I have used The Shower Massage, by Teledyne Water Pik.

PLASTIC SHOWER CAPS — These are indispensable for conditioning treatments, applying color glazes and as plain old shower caps. You can buy them in bulk from your beauty supply.

PLASTIC HAIR CLIPS -These are the hinged plastic clips used by hairdressers to section your hair when curling or rolling. You can either buy the kind that have little zig zag teeth or the type that look like long hair clips. If you get the kind with the teeth, you'll have to take care so you don't rip out your hair with the clip. These are great to use when you're texturizing your hair or separating into sections for conditioning.

BARRETTES, HEADBANDS, ETC. -Again, if I were select- ing these items for **my** hair, I'd stay away from plastic barrettes with metal clasps and plastic headbands with the tiny sharp plastic teeth. The metal barrette clasps give you that gradual, free hair cut and the headbands will help rake away what's left.

BETTER CHOICES: The plastic barrettes with no metal parts are best. Barrettes with a plastic "cover" and a little "stick" that pokes through are much kinder to our hair. Headbands whose undersides are covered with a smooth material like suede or grosgrain ribbon are better. Or you can fashion your own with a pretty silk or satin scarf. If you love putting your hair up in a chignon or bun, check out decorative **hair sticks**. You can find fancy ones in beauty supply stores or accessory boutiques or you can pick up lacquered Japanese chopsticks at import stores. Be imaginative!

FABRIC PONYTAIL HOLDERS — The elasticized terry cloth ponytail rings are popular but if your hair is kinky or extremely curly I recommend that you avoid them. In fact, they're not good for African hair period. What happens is that the loops and curls in unprocessed hair catches in the loops of the terry cloth and the absorbent quality of the material helps dry and break off processed hair. After all, terry cloth is used in towels and towels are designed to absorb moisture.

BETTER CHOICE: Use the type of holders made of a satin or silky type material with an elastic band sewn up inside. If you sew, you can make these yourself using silk or satin remnants. Simply sew a tube, run elastic through it as if you were making a casing and sew the casing ends into a circle.

PONYTAIL HOLDERS AND BANANA CLIPS — Make sure the plastic teeth and spaces in between them don't have razor sharp edges. The banana clips that have very low teeth should be checked for sharp edges also.

BETTER CHOICE: Generally, the holders and clips with widely spaced teeth are best for our hair.

ROLLERS — Get rid of your sponge rollers. The sponge's surface absorbs oil and moisture from your hair, which dries it out. The sponge's tiny plastic bubbles have edges that chew away at your hair. Velcro rollers, which stick to your hair and pull it out, should be banned. Ditto for brush rollers.

BETTER CHOICE: For wet sets, use flexible tube rollers or the smooth plastic type with holes. Make sure the tube rollers are of good quality and not simply wire covered by a glorified sponge roller. And don't sleep in rollers if you want hair.

LUBRICANTS AND HAIRDRESSINGS

There are different grades of lubricants and the proportion of oil and water will determine how your hair will respond. A pretty good way to test the consistency of a hair dressing or lubricant is to rub a dab onto the back of your hand and let it soak in for a few minutes. If you can, take a small section of hair and rub a little on the ends. If it's a cream dressing and it disappears without a trace then that's generally the way it will react on your hair.

POMADES are generally heavier with an ointment-type consistency. There are lots of pomades on the market — they range from the old standby, Dixie Peach Pomade, to Aveda's Shine, a humectant pomade that encourages curls. Generally, the glycerine-based, water soluble pomades are lighter and less greasy. Pomade is good for slicked down styles and waves. They add shine too.

CREAM HAIRDRESSINGS contain more water than pomades. They add shine, help moisturize and counteract brittleness. Some cream dressings seem to disappear into the hair and may not feel as lubricating as oilier dressings do. But if you like a light hairdressing, a creme may be right for you. Dab a bit on your hand to see how wet it's going to be. EXAMPLES: Vitapointe, DuSharme Haircreme.

STANDARD HAIRDRESSINGS are good for lubricating the ends of your hair. Their consistency is medium weight, lighter than a pomade. Use sparingly or your hair will have that greasy look and you'll have to wash it out. EXAMPLES: Ultra Sheen, Posner's Bergamot, VO5, etc.

OIL LOTIONS add moisture, oil and counteract brittleness. Since they do have a bit of water in them, I like to use it on my towel dried hair after shampooing and my hair absorbs it while I'm twisting or wet-setting. EXAMPLES: Luster's Pink Oil Moisturizer, AllWays Natural Hair Moisturizing Lotion.

GEL HAIRDRESSINGS are designed for control and shine, rather than lubrication. The ingredients include glycerine and water. EXAMPLES: Pre-Con Conditioning Sheen by Summit, Let's Jam! Shining and Conditioning gel by Attitudes Unlimited, Luster's Pink Oil Moisturizer Conditioning Shining Gel With Style Control.

MOISTURIZERS—I'm referring to moisturizing hair creme type preparations, *not* the stuff designed to "re-moisturize" hair that has been curly permed or "dry" curly permed. Moisturizers usually contain some sort of humectant (an ingredient that attracts and binds moisture in the air to your hair). They counteract brittleness and will sometimes enhance curl, depending upon how naturally kinky your hair is. Many of these preparations can be used as a traditional rinse out, after-shampoo conditioner or a hairdressing. EXAMPLE: Nexxus Humectress

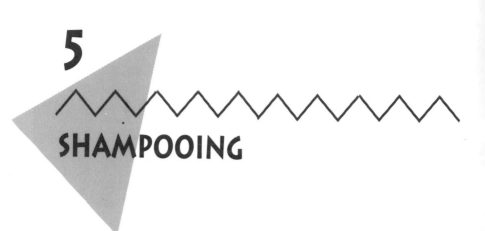

5

SHAMPOOING

The point of a shampoo is to clean your scalp and then your hair, in that order. I grew up on shampoo commercials featuring a willowy blonde with a creamy cap of suds covering waist-length hair. To let the shampoo companies tell it, you just pile your hair on top of your head and work those suds through...

Then there's reality. Try piling African hair on top of your head and working the suds through and you'll end up with a mess. And special care must be taken with chemically straightened hair, which can snap like limp spaghetti when wet.

So, here are some things to know about shampooing.

HOW TO CHOOSE A SHAMPOO

First , look for a shampoo that is pH balanced. pH is a measure of the degree of alkalinity or acidity in the product. A pH of around 5 is close to that of your hair and scalp, most shampoo labels specify whether or not it is pH balanced. If the shampoo is too alkaline, the cuticles of your hair will be open and it will feel coarser and tangle easier.

Choose a mild shampoo that won't strip every bit of natural oil from your scalp. Shampoos with egg, avocado and a lot of exotic vegetble and mineral additives do more for the promotion of the product that they do for your hair. I've tried baby shampoo, but found it very drying. I don't know why.

If you wear your hair unprocessed or in a style that plays off its natural texture, you'll probably discover that mild shampoos will make your hair more manageable.

▶ **Natural hair**—Gentle shampoo that minimizes dryness. Look for moisturizing shampoos.

▶ **Chemically straightened hair**—Gentle shampoos for chemically treated hair are fine. Look for moisturzing shampoos with protein.

▶ **Permanently colored hair**—Look for something mild, low in alkalinity and with lots of moisturizing qualities. *Special note* : Build-up remover shampoos — These shampoos will remove build up of styling products, hard water or other dulling, drying residues. These are good to use before coloring your hair because the color will "grab" better. They are also good if you've been doing a lot of swimming in chlorinated pools or the ocean. In fact, it's not a bad idea to use a build-up remover shampoo once a month or once every two months as a regular thing — but *always* be sure and use a good conditioner afterward.

DANDRUFF

If you think you have dandruff, examine your scalp and be sure that it isn't something a doctor should tend to. If you have severe, heavy flaking and itching, with reddened scalp or pus, you should see a dermatologist. If you have mild to moderate flaking, use a dandruff shampoo. There are several formulas on the market. Read labels carefully especially if you have processed hair.

Keratolytic shampoos have sulfur or salicylic acid. This chemical dissolves the hair flakes. Unfortunately, sulfur stinks so you will have an odor in your hair (remember Sulfur 8?) unless the label says otherwise.

Important — Don't use keratolytic shampoos with sulfur or salicylic acid if you have chemically texturized or chemically straightened hair — you'll be dreadfully sorry. Your hair will mat up into a tangled lump that is impossible to get out and the hair that is left will break right off.

Cystostatic shampoos contain tar, selenium sulfide, zinc pyrithione or pyrithione zinc. These ingredients slow down the cell turnover that creates flakes. They can also be drying and sometimes you scalp will overcompensate and over-produce oil. The tar shampoos will discolor your hair if it's been lightened or bleached. Again, read those labels!!!

The only shampoos I avoid are those which contain balsam. Now, I know this will cause a debate amongst you ladies who swear by the detangling properties of a certain brand of creamy balsam shampoo. Balsam is a resin that dries to a hard, clear film on the hair shaft. It feels good while you're washing, but it makes your hair drier later.

▶ How to prepare an inexpensive pre-shampoo treatment that will help keep your hair from drying out.

If your hair is dried out due to natural wear and tear or too many heated styling aids (we're going to work on that...) then you'll benefit from a hot oil treatment before shampooing. Your hair shafts will absorb the oil and the shampoo will clean your hair without stripping it dry.

Part your hair into three or four manageable sections. Warm up about a quarter cup of olive oil or the conditioning oil of your choice (see conditioning chapter for suggestions). You can heat the oil in the microwave, on the stove or put a dish of it in a pan of hot water, but be sure and test the temperature before putting it in your hair.

Part your hair into manageable sections. Use a cotton pad to pat the oil onto the ends of your hair. Work the oil up your hair shafts, section by section. Don't put the oil on your scalp.

Cover your hair with a plastic shower cap or plastic wrap. If you have time, wrap a towel over the plastic cap and let the heat from your head give you the treatment. Or sit under a bonnet dryer or heating cap for 20 minutes.

▶ How to shampoo without tangling your hair.

If your hair is longer than four inches, use plastic clips to separate it into three or four sections before shampooing. I prefer to wash my hair in the shower because I can rinse more thoroughly. Wet a section of hair and apply a quarter sized dollop of shampoo. Work it through the section with the pads of your fingers. Work your fingers through your hair and scalp in *one direction* and you'll minimize tangling and matting. Washing your hair in sections makes it easier to get to your scalp and concentrate on loosening the dead scalp cells without hopelessly matting and tangling your hair in the process.

Rinse each section for at least one minute and clip it out of the way. Finish your hair with a cool rinse.

It may take one to three latherings to feel clean but you don't have to clean until it squeaks. The exception to this is if you use a build-up remover shampoo. Build-up removers tend to give you that squeaky clean feel.

If your hair is very long, apply the shampoo to your scalp area only and work the suds down to the ends. Remember, the ends of your hair are drier and more porous and it doesn't take much to clean them or dry them out.

Now you're ready to condition.

6

CONDITIONING

It took me years to realize that conditioners are not miracle cures for abused hair. I bought a lot of stuff, mainly going by what friends said and whatever my hairdresser was pushing that month. I had a cabinet filled with rejects. You name it, I've probably bought it.

My expensive lesson taught me that the best conditioning treatment is preventive — preventing damage to your hair in the first place. Then you won't have to hope conditioners will repair the impossible. I've gone into a bit of detail to describe conditioners because I'd like to help you avoid learning the expensive way. In general, the purpose of conditioning your hair is to compensate for the daily wear and tear it takes. It's like moisturizing your skin after washing it — if you don't do it, you notice ashiness. Your hair needs the same type of after-shampoo care.

FOR HAIR BEYOND REPAIR,
Fried, dyed, falling out on the sides...

If your hair has been overprocessed or suffered severe heat damage, the only thing conditioners can do is to help stave off the inevitable — yes, cutting or a <u>serious</u> trim — until you can psychologically handle the loss. I know there are some products out there that claim they can repair your hair and I have used them. But if your hair is shot and you continue to abuse it — with heated styling appliances, chemicals, permanent coloring — conditioners won't save it. Sooner or later, the real you, broken ends and all, will be revealed. Believe me, I can talk about hair loss from personal experience.

SO, WHAT CAN CONDITIONERS DO?

Shampooing raises the hair's cuticle and when the roughened cuticles come in contact with each other, the hair tangles. You can compensate for this by acidifying your rinse water with a little lemon juice or vinegar, or using very cool water. But when your hair has been processed, conditioners are the only way to smooth the cuticle so you can comb your hair without tearing it out.

Some conditioners can help moisturize by replacing oils washed away by shampoos before smoothing the shingles down, creating a healthier appearance. In fact, hair that has been relaxed, texturized or permanently colored has raised shingles, even when it hasn't been shampooed. So it's important to condition, condition, condition!

Conditioners can also add body and volume to limp or thin hair. Here are the basic types of conditioners and what they do:

CREME RINSES AND FINISHING RINSES — In general, these rinses are used to detangle hair, by smoothing the cuticle and making it easier to comb. If you want to use them to control bushiness, you can double or triple the amount the manufacturer recommends. You don't need to spend a lot of money — the standard brands will do.

INSTANT CONDITIONERS—Instant conditioners smooth the hair's cuticle and detangle, but the also protect the hair shaft with a thin coating of hydrolized protein. Instant conditioners usually stay in your hair for one to three minutes and manufacturers will offer different formulas for different hair types.

DEEP CONDITIONERS AND PROTEIN CONDITIONERS — Deep conditioners give you a more intense conditioning treatment because they seal in moisture and coat the hair shaft with proteins. Most are left on for twenty or thirty minutes, with or without heat, then rinsed out. There are several types of proteins that are commonly used to beef up conditioning treatments, usually derived from animal or vegetable materials. The proteins are usually processed so they can enter the cuticle and cortex to *temporarily* replace keratin lost through heat or chemical damage.

RECONSTRUCTING CONDITIONERS — These contain complex proteins or nucleic acids that temporarily bond to the protein structure in your hair. Some heavy duty professional formulas can be thick and syrupy and you usually use a plastic cap and heat to activate the conditioner for at least 30 minutes before rinsing it out.

NOTE: You should be extremely careful when using the syrupy formulas because they can dry into a stiff helmet on your hair and must be rinsed out thoroughly or you can risk hair loss.

HAIR REPAIR CONDITIONERS—These generally have a thin, watery consistency and are "leave-in" conditioners. They're usually used for several consecutive shampoos and then your hair shaft remains "repaired". Many of these contain a formaldehyde-based ingredient called Formalin. If you're sensitive to formaldehyde (for instance, it is commonly used in nail polishes) you should avoid these conditioners.

CONDITIONING OILS

ROSEMARY OIL is distilled from the herb Rosemary, the herb you use on pork roasts. It is supposed to remove tangles and make your hair more manageable. I bought a small vial of the stuff — it's inexpensive— and tried it. It's touted as a daily grooming aid, but when I uncapped it, the smell rushed out and knocked me back! It's extremely odiferous; kinda like Sulfur 8 hairdressing — everyone will know you're using it. It didn't help remove tangles all that much either. It also has alcohol in it, which can be drying. If you try it and you feel it helps, fine, but I'd only recommend using it as a pre-shampoo treatment <u>only.</u>

COCONUT OIL is rather rich and usually fragrant, although I've purchased pure coconut oil form an herbal pharmacy and it didn't have much of a frangrance. If you're on vacation in Mexico, the Caribbean or most beach resorts, local vendors often hawk coconut oil for a couple of dollars. Instead of frying your skin with it, buy some and use it for an inexpensive , natural hot oil hair treatment right there on the beach.

JOJOBA OIL is the wonder oil that's very popular to put in hair care products. It's supposed to be a good skin moisturizer. I haven't tried it on my face but it seems to work okay on my hair. For as much as it costs —I paid almost five dollars for two ounces — it didn't do as much as I thought it was going to do. One manufacturer even recommends using it as an aftershave ...What the heck, if you've got the bucks, most health food stores have the jojoba.

OLIVE OIL, in my experience, is the most reasonable oil to use for conditioning. You can buy it at the supermarket, so it's easy to get. It costs about three or four dollars for a 25 ounce bottle. You don't need to use expensive virgin olive oil; plain, everyday olive oil will do.

CASTOR OIL is used in a lot of hairdressings marketed to men. It did an adequate job lubricating the ends of my hair, but I found castor oil to be kind of sticky and difficult to shampoo out. It also made my scalp flake.

HOW TO GET MAXIMUM BENEFIT FROM CONDITIONERS

▶ LEARN TO READ LABELS. You don't have to be a chemist to understand that if you see two conditioners whose main ingredient is hydrolyzed protein and one costs $15 and the other $5, that you're paying more when you probably don't have to .

▶ STOCK UP ON DISPOSABLE PLASTIC CAPS from your beauty supply and use them for conditioning treatments. In a pinch, use plastic kitchen wrap.

▶ USE A HEATING CAP to help your hair absorb deep conditioners and hot oil treatments. I bought mine at a beauty supply store several years ago and it still keeps my hair together.

▶ MINIMIZE OR ELIMINATE THE USE OF HEAT TO STYLE YOUR HAIR. If you don't have heat damage, you won't need to deep condition so often.

▶ DON'T LEAVE CONDITIONERS ON LONGER THAN

THE MANUFACTURER RECOMMENDS. If you leave it on longer, your hair will become limp and develop a coating that makes it hard to style. Your hair can only absorb so much material and the rest will sit on top of the hair shaft.

▶ **ALWAYS CONCENTRATE ON THE ENDS OF YOUR HAIR** because it's the oldest and driest part. So if you're running out of conditioner, be smart and use that last precious dab on your ends. The hair closest to your scalp is usually the healthiest unless you've been blasting it with heat or chemicals.

Since I occasionally texturize my hair once or twice a year, I always condition each time I shampoo. I give myself a hot oil treatment before shampooing. After shampooing, I'll use a moisturizing conditioner which doubles as a detangler. When my hair needs deep conditioning, I use a penetrating protein conditioner. Sounds like a lot, but I don't have a problem with brittle ends.

7

DAILY MAINTENANCE OR HOW TO KEEP YOUR HAIR FROM BREAKING OFF

If you are diligent about the way you treat your hair physically, in addition to avoiding the use of heated appliances or at worst severely minimizing the use of heat, you will prevent 95 percent of hair loss due to breakage. I know this is true because I've done it and have the hair to prove it. I have even made the mistake of over-straightening my hair and due to the way I handled it and avoided blow drying and other heat, I managed to grow it out **and** keep the length. I was then able to gradually trim away the damaged hair **without** a major haircut. I learned then that my hair looked and felt better with little or no chemical straightening.

Let me stress that this isn't about having **long** hair as it is about having **healthy** looking, full hair.

Hair maintenance is quite simple when you think about it. They are probably things that you have heard most of your life but when you see pictures of the latest weave you toss caution out the window and do anything you can to get that long, shiny look. But you're about to learn better.

After shampooing and conditioning, there are some other things that you need to do to your hair to keep it supple. Here they are:

HOW TO COMB AND DE-TANGLE

First of all, you can't comb your hair properly if you haven't gotten the tangles out. Here's how you do it:

DE-TANGLING: Always work from the ends of your hair toward your scalp. If your hair is natural or texturized, use a spritz of water on the section you are trying to de-tangle. The water softens the hair and makes it easier to work with. In fact, I prefer to comb my hair only when it is dampened. You can also use a dab of cream rinse or moisturizing conditioner to help it along.

COMBING: After you've de-tangled, part your hair into three or four sections. Then, use your wide-toothed comb and gently, but firmly comb through. If you reach a snag, stop and de-tangle with your fingers, don't be impatient and jerk the comb through.

TIP: You'll find that if you wear your hair naturally or texturized in a curly or wavy style you will tend to use your fingers for everyday combing and use the comb when you are changing styles — let's say from crimps to a traditional straight wet set. If you're wearing it curly or natural, fingers will preserve more curls than a comb.

SHEDDING: If you take out snarls with your fingers instead of the comb, most or all of the hair that comes out will be shed hair. By this I mean hair that has completed it's growth cycle and fallen from the follicle. Hair that have been shed naturally have a little whitened end from the dead root. Of course, if you're shedding an unusually large amount of hair you should see a doctor.

I know a lot of you will say "That isn't right! That's unclean! you've got to comb your hair with a comb every day!" Well, I'm here to tell and show you, with shoulder-length proof, that keeping your hair tangle-free has nothing to do with raking a comb through it three times a day. Girlfriends, forget those shampoo commercials!

HOW TO BRUSH PROPERLY

First, get your **gentle**, natural bristle brush (see "Tools of the Trade").

The point of brushing is to distribute scalp oils and brush away loose scales, right? But if you have curly, kinky hair, you can't pull the brush through to the ends of your hair without tearing some hair out. So first, de-tangle your hair, then part your hair to the scalp and brush from the part, out to the ends. If it helps, part your hair into three or four large sections and then part and brush each section. You don't have to do this every single day; just like you

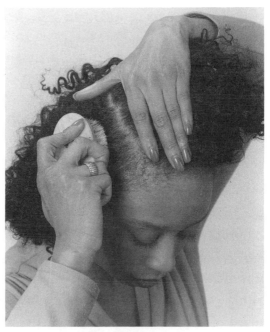

How to brush your hair and have some left to style afterward

wouldn't need to exfoliate your facial skin every day. Remember, what you are doing is stimulating your scalp, distributing oils and loosening sloughed off cells.

I know a lot of you have been told you must brush your hair every day, but if your hair is delicate and curly you will simply tear it out. Try thoroughly brushing once a week and substituting scalp massage between brushings. It's also a good idea to brush thoroughly before you shampoo. If you're still unconvinced, save your old, hard nylon brush filled with hair and compare it to your gentler brush after two weeks of my method.

HOW TO MASSAGE YOUR SCALP

Put your hands under your hair , with the pads of your fingers—not your fingernails—resting on your scalp. Using your fingers in back and forth and circular motions, knead your scalp with your fingers. Spread open your hands, press your palms against your scalp and contract your hand. Concentrate on having your fingerpads maintain contact with your scalp and you won't tangle your hair. If you're doing your own massage, you can part and pin your hair into three or four large sections and massage each part separately to ensure that you won't tangle it. Scalp massage is much more pleasurable if you can get a friend to do it for you, but make sure they know how to do it correctly. It's better to do it yourself than end up with a bunch of knots in your hair. Or you can pick up an electric, hand-held scalp massager at a discount appliance store. It feels great and you don't have to spend a fortune.

DON'T SLEEP IN ROLLERS — They contribute to hair breakage. Protect your hair while you sleep. Use a satin pillowcase, pillow cover or wrap your hair in a silk or satin scarf.

8

THE GREAT ESCAPE: GETTING OUT FROM UNDER A PERM

Okay. There are two ways to eliminate a chemical straightener or overprocessed hair.

✂ Cutting it off.

✂ Growing it out and gradually trimming it away.

We'll get into the pros and cons of each method, suggestions on how to grow out of a perm and I'll tell you how I got out of my straightener.

CUTTING IT OFF — ADVANTAGES.

It gets you to the promised land quicker. No doubt about it. In my experience, this is the most graceful way to get out of a perm. You'll become acquainted with the real you. People will consider you to be beautifully Afrocentric, interesting, stylish, sensual. You will have a very carefree hair care regimen — you can shampoo, condition and go! You can wear chic hats, beautiful earrings. You can now feel sorry for the permed women who have to spend precious party time in the bathroom, trying to pat their limp and matted hairdo's into something presentable. With the money you'll save on hair repair and despair, you can concentrate on good skin care and your face will be radiant. For the first time in your life, you won't care what the weather is like. You can live at the beach or use the pool at the gym to tone up your body — swimming, for those of you who haven't been informed, is the best exercise because it works **everythang.** And for those of you who are really concerned about the brothers' reaction —don't be. There are **plenty** of brothers who like a chic, cropped natural 'do on a good looking sister. Trust me. The ones you get flak from ain't worth the aggravation.

CUTTING IT OFF — DISADVANTAGES

You'll probably have to put up with a lot of remarks from friends and relatives at first, but they'll get used to it. If you are cutting your hair to grow it out long and natural, they'll be envious once you start strutting your new, **strong, long,**

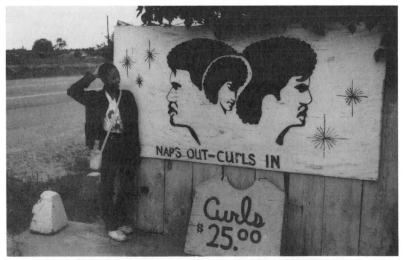

My escape from the perm in Mound Bayou, Mississippi,
where the Jheri curl reigned supreme.

thick stuff. Even the friends who don't say much of anything are gonna notice an improvement. There's no way you can stand a head of strong, thick natural looking hair next to a chemically straightened, hot curled or gelled down head of hair and not come out looking superior and desirable.

Some men have strange ideas about women who have short natural hair. That's their problem and you have to be woman enough to do what is good for you because that's the only way you're going to be good enough for anyone else. The person who truly cares about you is going to see that.

GROWING IT OUT — ADVANTAGES.

If you really can't handle cutting it off, or you have not been blessed with a well shaped head or nice hairline, growing it out and gradually cutting it off is the way to do it. But please don't confuse this point — the overprocessed/chemically straightened hair has to go and the sooner, the better.

GROWING IT OUT — DISADVANTAGES

You will have to contend with two radically different textures of hair. This means extreme diligence. Those of you who hate dealing with even a little new growth on your bone straight perm will find this aspect very hard to deal with. Imagine a couple inches of the real, natural you underneath four or five inches of bone straight hair. The hair will snap off where the two extreme textures meet — breakage can be delayed but it's inevitable. Breakage and bondage to rollers are the ultimate disadvantages with a bone straight perm. Also keep in mind that with two distinctly different textures, your hair will react in two distinctly different ways to heat, humidity, funky hot dance clubs etc.

MY CHOICE — COLD TURKEY

I cut my hair off to 1/2 an inch in 1988. My husband loved it because it no longer took two hours before I was ready to go out. I could go swimming and to the beach and ride with the car windows down. I wore baaaad hats and neat, exotic earrings. I didn't wear rollers to bed anymore and my husband could run his fingers through my little kinky curls as much as he wanted without me complaining that my hair was messed up. He also revealed that my natural hair **felt** better to the touch than the chemically straightened hair. He gave me toe tingling shampoos in the bathtub and in the shower. He had always wanted to shampoo my hair for me, but I wouldn't let him because I didn't want him to mat up my perm.

With relatives and friends it was a different story. Right after I cut my hair, we visited relatives in Tennessee who hadn't seen me for years. And there I was, practically bald as far as they were concerned. One aunt told me she "sure would be glad when my hair came back." The other aunt said something about "if that's what I liked I should be happy but it certainly wasn't for her and what did my mother think about this?" My mother and father couldn't wait for my hair to grow back. My friends generally didn't comment too much, figuring it was yet another hair episode.

When my hair grew out my husband and most people loved it. The Nappy Hair Phobia people went into their "long and straight" campaign and are waiting (in vain) for me to "get my hair done." But the best feeling was when my aunts saw me two years later they were touching my thick ponytail and asking "Is it **all** yours?" And it really makes my day when people work up enough nerve to ask me if I have a weave or hair extensions.

GROWING OUT OF A PERM—WAYS AND MEANS

NOTE : There is a difference between chemically straightened or permed hair and texturized hair. A texturizer is a mild chemical relaxer applied so that it relaxes a little of the natural curl, while leaving your hair kinky and curly. Since texturized hair (when done properly) is very close to the texture of natural African hair, you don't have the problems associated with chemically straightened hair.

▶ **TRIM** at least 1/2 an inch of hair per month.

▶ **USE STYLING METHODS THAT REQUIRE LITTLE OR NO HEAT.** This includes the traditional wet sets or the wrap, but you should know that the effectiveness of both these methods will only last a maximum of two to three months. Later on, try the Corkscrew Crimp which will help disguise the difference in textures.

▶ **BE EXTRA, EXTRA CAREFUL WHEN HANDLING YOUR HAIR.** This is very important. Your hair is at its most vulnerable when it has two radically different textures. You'll spend more time de-tangling with your fingers than ever. You can no longer comb or brush straight through your hair or you will have breakage on an everyday basis. You'll also need to sleep in silk or satin scarves. Review the chapter on "Daily Maintenance."

▶ **BEWARE** of using a "warm comb" or curling iron to touch up new growth. The amount of heat necessary to relax strong virgin regrowth is going to be too much for your weaker, bone straightened hair. One of the textures will snap under the stress and heat. Guess which one?

▶ **USE STYLES THAT EMPHASIZE CURLS INSTEAD OF SLEEKNESS.** Remember, go with nature, not against it.

▶ **USE BRAID EXTENTIONS**—preferably cornrows for a couple months, until you have enough new growth —a couple inches — to work with. Try to remember that the braid extentions are a **transitional** tool, not a substitute for hair.

▶ **IF YOU DECIDE THAT YOU JUST CAN'T LIVE WITH-OUT THE PERM,** consider having a short perm. It is much easier to manage a short chemically straightened style without heat. But I hope you'll give natural or at least texturized hair an honest shot.

9

WANTED: MO' BETTA HAIR

By now, some of you might be thinking, "I really don't need to know all this stuff. That's what I pay a hairdresser for." Well, if you don't know what time it is **before** you step into the salon, you might end up wishing for a magician instead of a beautician.

I'll be happy to testify to this.

I happened to work with two African-American women who'd had their hair texturized. Texturizing is using a chemical straightener to slightly relax our excessively loopy curls, so that the curls are simply stretched a little, instead of being ironed out straight. (See Page 98 for more information on texturizing.)

One woman's hair was cut short in a curly cap with shorter sides and nape. There were little curls all over and they looked very natural. She said she used a little gel and a little curl activator sometimes, but she didn't have a curly perm or jheri curl. She said her hairdresser had put a relaxer on her hair for a few minutes and rinsed it out. This, I had to try. I made an appointment with her hairdresser — I'll call him "Mr. Bill" —and told him I wanted the same thing.

I had a little more length than she did, so I told Mr. Bill I wanted it cut into a bob, or wedge and texturized. He looked at my hair and kept repeating "bob" like it was a foreign dialect. He said I'd need a curly perm, a jheri curl to achieve a curly look. I explained again that I simply wanted it texturized, I wanted the relaxer in just long enough to release my natural curl and then rinsed out, just like my friend's. He swore that wouldn't work on my hair and that the jheri curl would give me the look I wanted. What he was really saying, was that my hair was too kinky, too nappy to simply be texturized.

I let him do it.

Although this man had never seen me or my hair before that day, he didn't bother with a strand test to see how my hair would react to the chemicals. He just commenced with the curly perm. For those of you who haven't had the pleasure of a jheri curl, here's a quick review of the process. A thioglycolate solution (the same solution used to permanently curl Caucasian hair) is used to prestraighten kinky hair before it's wrapped around perm rods. After the hair is rodded, the thio is rinsed out and the hair is saturated with waving solution. Then you put on a plastic cap and sit under a dryer, periodically saturating your hair with waving solution, until your hair curls by itself. The whole process takes a few hours.

After my hair was done, Mr. Bill snipped off about 3/4 inch of overprocessed hair. Then he soaked it with the standard curl activator and moisturizer.

Voila! I had the same old tight, greasy scary curl I'd seen coming and going. No bob. No natural looking curlicues, no nothing. I walked out in a disgusted daze.

The jheri curl was one of the worst, if not **the** worst hair mistakes I have ever made. My hair was so overprocessed that after it was shampooed, it was like a dry brillo pad. I'd almost say it was the texture of pubic hair, but pubic hair is softer and has more body. I wish I were exaggerating, but I kid you not. It drank bottles of activator. My husband just shook his head and avoided touching it. Folks who used to have plenty to say to me, got real quiet or avoided the subject of hair altogether. I put in a supply of headbands — the style LaToya Jackson made popular for a while — to try and disguise the fact that it was a jheri curl. I was one headband-and-scarf wearing woman. When my mother-in-law, who is a cosmetologist, suggested I sleep with a plastic shower cap over my head to keep the moisture in, I threw up my hands in defeat. I ran back to braids until I could cut that mess off.

After I got rid of the hair ruined by the scary curl, I had about 1 1/2 inches left. It was so short, I'd cringe when it was hot combed. Another hairdresser helped me fashion a 'do that my husband christened "The Mia," named after the ultra short, brushed to the front 'do that actress Mia Farrow had in the movie "Rosemary's Baby." I thought Mia's hair was fierce, but I hated my version, and couldn't wait for it to grow out.

When my hair grew out to somewhere around chin-length, I sought out the services of another hairdresser. I wanted liberation from the hot comb needed to maintain my 'do, so I asked the other texturized lady for a hairdresser reference.

I told the hairdresser —"Missy" for short— that I wanted the same thing my girlfriend had. Missy relaxed my hair - with more attention to how my hair processed —and let it dry naturally. She told me how my hair would have that natural wave. It was gonna have that natural body. It was gonna be **fierce**. She worked a little gel and curl activator in

A hair "don't" in my Cavalcade of Hairstyles

my locks and explained how I could get that curly look by using my hands and hair tools instead of blow dryers. When my hair was wet, it had that loosely waved look of wet Caucasian hair so I figured it would dry like that too.

But that didn't happen. Once again, my hair had been overprocessed. I added the gel and scrunched in the waves, just like Missy showed me, but it did little to enhance it. It had that look that white girls with overprocessed hair had — limp and frizzy, with parts that were bone straight. Missy told me this would pass once I got the hang of handling my hair.

When I premiered my new 'do at work, my boss asked if I'd gone swimming on my lunch break. Colleagues figured it was yet another episode in my Cavalcade of Hairstyles.

After a while, I noticed my hair looked thinner and shorter. This was caused by the overprocessing, but I didn't know enough to realize that. Missy told me that if I cut one side of my hair noticeably shorter than the other, it would grow back thicker. I wanted hair so bad that I did it.

It didn't work. I just looked lopsided.

After a few weeks, I figured that a short style would work better with my "slightly relaxed" hair. I envisioned a 'do with short sides and a curly top with tendrils framing my face. A gamine look, a funky Anita Baker look, if you will.

Missy said I could achieve this look without rollers and blow dryers — another wash-n-go triumph.

What I got was another wet look, as in limp jheri curl. The only way I could get the chic short look I envisioned was with the help of a curling iron. That way, I could get the tendrils to frame my face and hide my hairline and forehead.

I did the curling iron hustle and I was very cute ... for a while. Then it began to grow out. It wasn't flowing down my back or anything, it was just that the new growth was screwing up my cut. I began using the curling iron as a combination curler and hair straightener.

Soon I was going to work with curling iron burns on the nape of my neck where the curling iron had kissed me. One morning I tried to straighten my wispy bangs and tendrils and it kissed me right in the middle of my forehead. There was no way to disguise it. Everyone knew I'd burned it with the curling iron. It was truly pitiful. There had to be a better way.

I went back to Missy and had her cut my hair off down to 1/2 an inch. That was in 1988 and I haven't been back to a hairdresser since.

SALON SURVIVAL

What's the moral of this story? What you **don't** know about your hair **can** hurt you. You should have a basic working knowledge of your hair, just like the rest of your body.

The hairdressers were not entirely responsible for my fiascoes. It was my responsibility to get up out of the chair, walk out of the salon and get another opinion before getting a service I had reservations about. But I also realize that when you consult a professional, you expect that he or she has some degree of expertise and you tend to take their advice.

On the other hand, Missy and Mr. Bill never did proper strand tests to see how the chemicals would work on my hair. Mr. Bill did an oral test, as in "do you have a relaxer in your hair?" Missy used my entire head as a test. Many hairdressers believe that because they have worked on many heads, they can tell how your hair is going to react to a chemical process simply by looking at it and touching it. An honest cosmetologist will tell you that *the only way to be sure* is to do a strand test. Differences in porosity, hair density, previous coloring or chemical alterations etc. — they all affect each person's hair differently and the only way to be sure is to test it.

Of course, my opinion is that it is better to avoid chemical straightening altogether and at the most, have a professional apply a slight, and I do mean slight, texturizer.

I know hairdressers who say testing takes too much time. If you were to ask these people for a strand test, some are apt to say "if you don't trust my judgement, then you can take your business somewhere else!" Take it from someone who has been there that you are better off doing so. I think it is better to risk momentary bitchiness from a stylist, than to have to walk into "People's Court" with a scarf on your head, explaining how you lost your hair and why you deserve a cash settlement.

I'd like to make it clear that I am not advocating a boycott of hair care professionals. I am simply saying that if you understand your hair and what is good for it as well as what is bad, then you can find a professional who can take care of you, not take advantage of you. Let's face it, unless you have big bucks and a live-in hairdresser, you're going to have to deal with your own hair between appointments anyway.

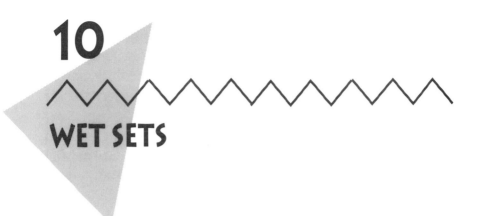

10

WET SETS

You're about to learn some ways to style natural and texturized African hair as well as how to deal with curls.

Most of you are probably turned off to wet sets because you think of them as being old fashioned. I had the same attitude. Once I learned how to use a blow dryer and electric curling iron, I kissed that so-called old stuff goodbye.

My appliance abuse began in college. I lived in a co-ed dorm — that is the men were segregated on one floor and women were on the rest. No one was gonna be caught dead in rollers. Now for white girls it was easy. They could get wash-n-wear perms or get up and work out with the hot rollers. Plus, it was cool to be caught in the laundry room in a skimpy nightie and slicked back wet hair with a few strategically placed tendrils falling over the forehead. Sexy, huh?

Not so for us. Unless you had naturally straight, wavy or loosely curled hair, your stuff was gonna draw up or puff up soon as it began to dry. That meant you had to commence to styling pretty soon after shampooing. You either stayed cloistered in your room and hoped nobody but girlfriends stopped by or you got hip and got some tools. That's how sisters who started the semester with thick, healthy, shoulder length hair ended it with transparent, collar-length hair by spring break.

If you or your parents had cash, you could make a weekly or bi-weekly pilgrimage to a hairdresser. My budget didn't quite cover a weekly hair appointment. But I **could** afford an electric curling iron and blow dryer. That was the beginning of the end of my hair.

I was too tired (too lazy) to come in after a late date and roll up my hair. And to be honest, roller sets were uncool. Everybody aimed for that bouncin' and behavin' look and you could only get that with a blow dryer or so we thought. Real rollers left marks. Curling irons gave you that smooth look. If your hair was on the short side — and mine always was— "bumping the ends" with a curling iron would preserve every last micro inch of your 'do.

There were sisters who maintained their manes throughout their undergraduate enrollment. But of course, being young and into hair immediacy, we just thought they'd been blessed with "good hair." What they'd been blessed with was someone who explained the fact of successful African hair care to them at an early age; constant heat and heavy chemicals don't mix. Add trying to keep up with every hair fad and you have a recipe for problems.

I've since discovered — through trial and error — that wet sets don't have to make you look like you're stuck in a time warp. You can adapt wet set techniques to your texturized hair. The biggest bonus? Wet sets last longer than styles that depend on curling irons or hot rollers.

THE NATURE OF CURLS

The most important thing to remember about styling curly hair is that there is strength in numbers. Notice that people with naturally curly hair have what appear to be ringlets. Ringlets are groups of curly hairs. When the ringlets are separated, the curls appear frizzy. That's because each curly strand stands separate from the rest.

When you brush extremely curly hair, it looks frizzy. You may have noticed that when women with naturally straight hair get curly permanents, stylists will use extremely wide toothed combs or even picks to style it. If they use brushes, the bristles are widely spaced. They are trying to prevent frizz.

Those of you who can remember how your unprocessed hair looks (and believe me, some of you haven't seen the natural you for years...) may have noticed that some of those African spirals will separate into little coils on their own. These spirals are really visible when your hair is damp or wet. Ladies, these are **curls**. If you comb or brush them, they may separate into frizz, depending upon the condition or natural texture of your hair.

Kinky, curly hair, by nature of its construction, is more delicate than naturally straight hair. You'll find that the curls soften when wet and they are easier to comb through. You'll also find that your fingers are the best tools for arranging your hair in curly styles.

Let me hip you to something else. You'll find that your hair will be infinitely more manageable when you style it in curly styles, even when you wet set it. I know we all like change every once in a while, but you'll soon see that you're fighting against nature by trying to go straight. But hey, you only live once, right?

SETTING AIDS

When setting the hair without using heat, it's usually best to start with freshly shampooed and conditioned, damp hair. If you don't want to go through all that, you can mist your hair with water and still get good results.

Remember, unless you have time to spare, the wetter your hair is, the longer it will take to dry. If you want to use a hair dryer, I recommend you invest in a bonnet-type dryer or one with a soft bonnet attachment. You can pick one of these up at a discount appliance store. These are gentler on your hair than a blow dryer and your hands are free to do other things.

Bonnet dryers are also good for applying transparent color glazes and deep conditioners. If you have dry skin, be sure and moisturize your face first.

▶ **TO GET THE BEST SET**, you must pull the hair taut enough so that it will stretch around itself or the roller and dry.

▶ **SET IT WET** with or without setting gel. A product I've had great success with is Miss Cool Five Minute Set by Soft Sheen Products. It comes in a creme formula for dry or pressed hair and in a lotion form. I find that the creme works well for the Corkscrew Crimp set (more on that in this chapter) and it also adds lubrication, which is always great for natural or texturized hair. The lotion formula is better for straight looks.

▶ **FOR QUICKER WET SETS**, towel blot your hair before dampening with setting aids or try one of the commerically prepared quick setting aids formulated for African hair.

▶ **TO REFRESH A SET BETWEEN SHAMPOOS**, lightly mist your hair before twisting or setting. If you saturate your hair, you'll have a longer drying time, which will tempt you to use heat.

THE CORKSCREW CRIMP SET

** Produces unusual waves that curl at the ends. What is unique about this style is that you can leave the curl bunches together for a curly "neo-dreadlock" look or sepa-

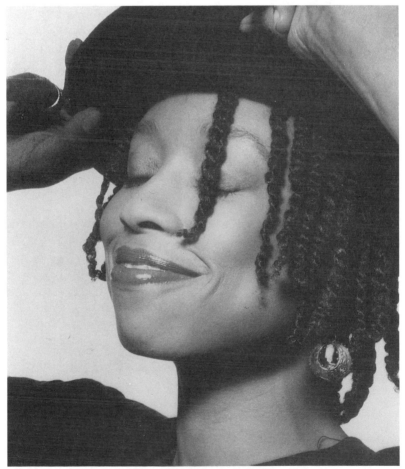

The Corkscrew crimp set
You won't be ashamed to be seen in public with these twists

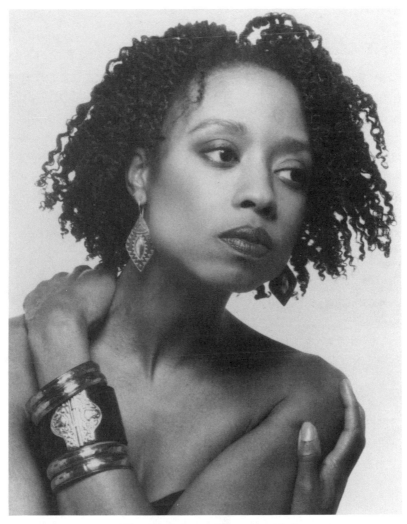

The Corkscrew crimp unveiled
This is shorter. . .

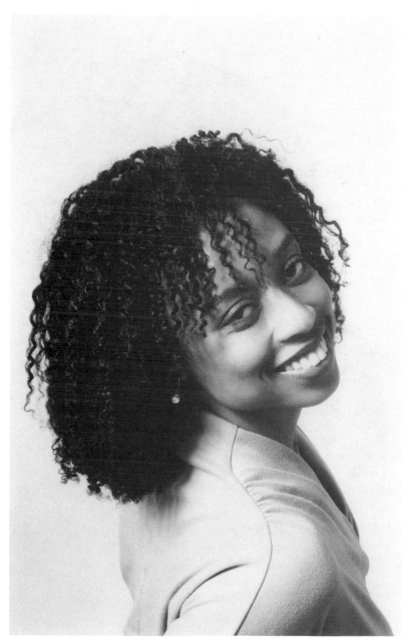

The Corkscrew crimp. . .
A little longer.

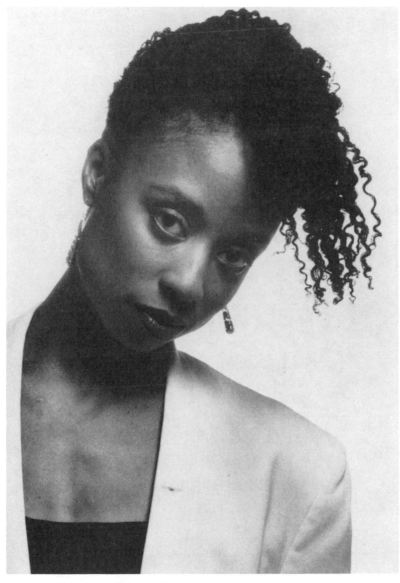

The Corkscrew crimp upsweep

rate them for a curly crimped look that people will assume is natural and pretty. It is extremely versatile, you can pin your hair into upsweeps or whatever you want.

This style can be a real head-turner. Many women stop, check me out and ask how they can get the look. They assume I've braided or crimped my hair, but they can't figure out how to get the natural looking curl at the ends. It's also a great way to have style and texture without using heat, so it's gentle and promotes breakage-free growth.

WHAT YOU NEED Spritz bottle, wide toothed comb, setting creme, clips or faux tortoiseshell hair pins to separate your hair into sections and your fingers. HOW TO SET You can wet your hair, part into one inch sections as if you were going to roll them in curlers. Instead, part the one-inch section into two sections and twist the two sections together. Twist down to the ends. If necessary, furl the ends around your fingers so that the hair twists onto itself. When your hair is dry, unfurl the twists with your fingers. To style, separate and arrange the waves with your fingers, do not comb or you will separate the curl bunches and your hair will simply frizz.

If your hair is very tightly curled, you might consider a mild texturizer. A texturizer slightly stretches out your natural kinks and curls without straightening it.

HOW TO MAINTAIN THE STYLE—If you sleep with a silk or satin scarf (short to medium length hair) or put it in a ponytail and sleep on a satin pillow cover, your crimps should last until your next shampoo. The more you separate the curl bunches, the more volume you'll get. I find that the closer my hair gets to shampoo time, the more voluminous and natural looking it gets. If you want it to look fresher between sets, you can mist the frizzy sections with a little water and setting creme and twist them up.

If you have the time, you can also give your hair a good brushing , twist it up again and sleep on it —you can sleep on twists without a scarf — take them out in the morning and go!

BONUS: You can be seen in public while your hair sets because you don't use unsightly rollers. If your twists are neatly done you can go bareheaded, which helps them dry faster, or wear a cute hat and let the twists peek out.

THE SHAKE

The Shake is another no roller, no heat styling method that works best on natural or texturized hair of any length. Depending upon the texture of your hair, you'll come out with a tiny neo dreadlock look or tiny spirals that are quite attractive. The Shake simply helps encourage your hair to separate into its natural curl bunches and spirals. It is a way of enhancing natural texture and promoting health and stress-free growth. It is also a good "wash-n-go" style.

WHAT YOU NEED Alcohol-free gel, lubricant of your choice and wet hair.

HOW TO SET Shampoo and condition. Take your gel and lubricant in the shower with you. Put a bit of lubricant in the palm of your hands and scrunch it into the ends of your hair. Then take the gel and do the same thing, but extend it to the roots of your hair as well. In other words, you're lubricating your ends and gelling everything else. Now, while your hair is fairly wet, just shake your head in all directions, letting the weight of the water help separate the spirals and coils into their own free form look. Get out of the shower and *lightly blot* excess water from your hair without disturbing the spirals and coils.

HOW TO STYLE Lightly pat into the shape you want and let dry. If your hair is cut into a short, tapered style you get a chic, natural look. If it is longer you'll get more of a free form, uninhibited look.

THE NEO JOSEPHINE

This is a great, no heat, roller free method of styling short to medium length hair. It is essentially a chic, slicked back look that looks best on natural or texturized hair because of the tiny waves it produces. Those with natural heads can also get this look with a bit of help.

WHAT YOU NEED Non-alcoholic gel, pomade or lubricant of your choice. Silk or satin scarf.

HOW TO SET Shampoo and condition your hair or dampen it with a spritz bottle. Lubricate the ends with your lubricant and work pomade or gel around the hairline and lightly through the rest of your hair. Smooth all your hair back from your face —with your fingers and palms — smooth it taut against your scalp. Tie the scarf gypsy-style over your head so it makes a smooth tight cap. Leave it on until your hair dries a bit. The scarf helps smooth your hairline and helps bring out the tiny pretty waves.

HOW TO STYLE If your hair is short and you have a nice hairline it can be very sexy. If your hair is longer, you can do a bun or small chignon. The Neo Josephine can also be used to tame hair into a single French braid or other styles that require a smooth look.

THE ZORRO SET

This set produces gentle zig-zag or z waves with little curly ends or waved ends, depending upon how you wrap the hair ends. It gives good looking waves that don't look "set". It works best on hair that is at least five inches or longer. If your hair is too short, you won't be able to wrap it around the rollers.

WHAT YOU NEED Flexible tube rollers, wide toothed comb, setting aid of your choice, spritz bottle. You can buy flexible tube rollers in different widths at beauty supply stores. Examine the quality before you buy; some of the cheaper brands are simply glorified sponge rollers with wire in the middle —you don't want those.

HOW TO SET Take a section of hair, the smaller the section, the curlier the look; for looser waves use slightly larger sections of hair. Remember, larger sections will take longer to dry. Bend the roller in half into a "U" shape and slip it onto a section of hair up to your scalp so the prongs of the "U" are facing downward. Then weave the hair in and out and around the prongs of the "U". Wrap the last inch or so around one of the prongs. Pull the hair ends taut when wrapping that last bit and it will stay wrapped. Twist the ends of the roller together. Let dry and unwrap carefully. If you want the waves to last, use your fingers rather than combing through.

The Zorro set dries quicker than conventional roller sets, even when you dry naturally. You can also use a blow dryer with a diffuser attachment if you want or a bonnet type dryer.

See Page 98 for more information on the "U" prong roller.

STEP 1
How to wrap a Zorro using "U" prong rollers

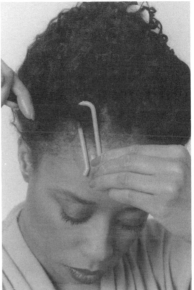

STEP 2
Just weave in and out

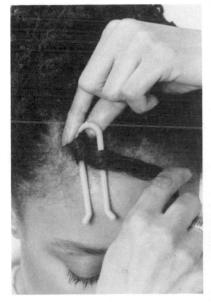

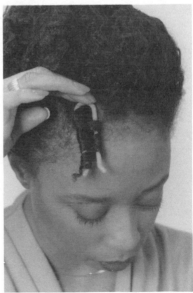

STEP 3
(you can also use flexible rubber tube rollers)

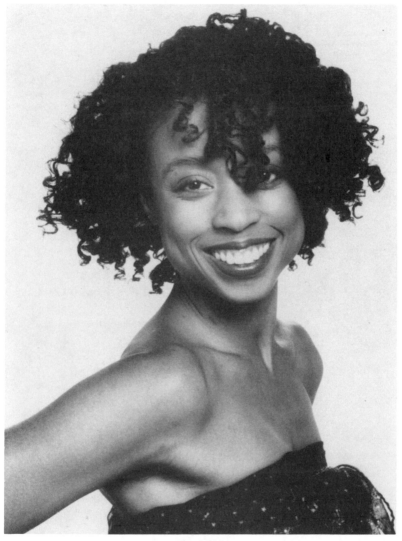

The Zorro
Mid length set on flexible tube rollers

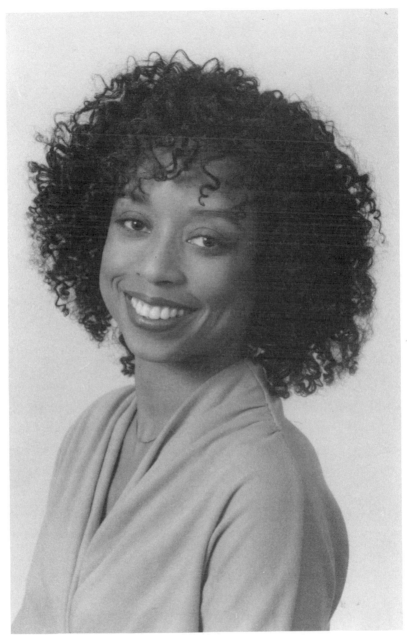

The Zorro
On longer hair, set on "U" prong rollers

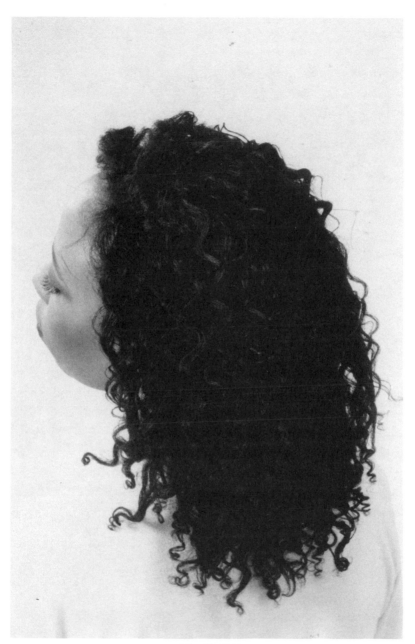

The Zorro
Even Longer—can be set on "u" prong or flexible tube rollers

THE WRAP

This is a great set for texturized or straightened hair because you can get a sleek look that's full of body without blow drying. No heated appliances means no heat related breakage. Therefore, if you have chronic breakage problems with your sides and back, devising styles that don't require much manipulation will allow them a little rest.

The big bonus? You don't have to sleep in rollers to maintain it because your head is used as a giant roller.

WHAT YOU NEED A liquid, non-alcoholic gel or "wrapping lotion" available at beauty supply stores.

HOW TO SET Start with wet hair. Slick the gel through your hair. Starting from whichever side you like, take small sections of hair and comb it across your forehead and as far around the back as it will go. Smooth it down at the ends and use a long wave clip to keep it in place.

Take another, small vertical section and wrap it around the section you just wrapped. Remove the clip from the previous section and smooth the new section over it. If the hair starts to pull away, dampen it with gel or wrapping lotion.

Keep wrapping and smoothing out wrinkles. If it gets hard to smooth out, just spritz with some water and smooth a bit of gel through. Spritz an end paper with a little water and smooth down any frizzy parts.

You should end up with a smooth cap of hair. If your hair is feathered toward your face, you should wrap so the ends frame the face.

Wrap your head with a silk scarf and sit under a dryer or let it air dry. Be sure it is completely dry before bushing or combing it out. You'll get a curvy, sleek look with lots of body.

IF YOU WANT HEIGHT IN THE CROWN of your hair, section off the crown into three or four sections, apply the gel and roll each section in the direction you want the crown to fall using plastic rollers. You should use the type that are smooth, with big holes — the kind for conventional sets.

TO MAINTAIN THE STYLE When you're ready to sleep, brush or comb your hair around your head as you did when you did the initial set and tie it with a silky scarf. That's it — that's The Wrap.

THE STRAIGHT LOOK

Also known as the conventional wet set. This is for those days when you feel you've got to conform or you just want a change. Straight wet sets can also be real hair savers during those times when you're tempted to give up all your hard work and get something "easier" — a straight permanent relaxer. Sometimes, all it takes to snatch you back into reality is dealing with straightened hair for a week. Remember? Not being able to stand a strong wind, wondering how to make it look decent when it's too short to make a bun or ponytail and you're too tired to curl it...

WHAT YOU NEED Good old traditional smooth plastic rollers with holes in them. You can try using large flexible tube rollers or perm rods but it takes **forever** to dry without using lots of heat. You'll also need a bonnet dryer.

HOW TO SET Part your hair into one inch sections or the size you want, depending upon the look you want. It works best when your hair is wet and you'll probably find that a traditional setting gel will help. Since wet hair is key to straight wet sets, spritz your hair if the section you're about to roll up, dries out.
The larger the roller the straighter the look.

11

DON'T LET YOUR HAIRSTYLE DICTATE YOUR LIFESTYLE

Before I enlightened myself, I used to make do with my chronically damaged hair and tried every new conditioner that came out, hoping for a quick fix. Nothing really worked until I gave my hair a rest and wore braids for a year and a half. Voila! My hair grew to shoulder length and I thought I was a star.

People who'd turned their noses up at my braids had plenty of compliments when they saw my straightened hair.

"Lonnice, it's gorgeous! I just love your hair!" The most popular refrain was "And it's really grown, hasn't it?"

I planned to debut my new hair at a party that weekend. It wasn't far from the beach and the fog rolled in early, so I fortified my do with a heavy dose of hair spray. The party was only a ten minute walk away, what could go wrong?

Soon as I hit the party, I made a beeline for the bathroom so I could prepare for my big entrance. When I looked in the mirror, I almost died. My satiny, blow-dried tresses had turned to cotton! The ends were fuzzy, the bangs I'd swept to the side stood up in a nappy salute, just like Buckwheat's. The only thing the hairspray did was hold my new helmet together. I pulled the stiff mess back into a ponytail and patted the bangs into the best shape I could. There was no way to disguise my 'do — I hadn't been there long enough to play it off as the result of some buck wild dancing. The heartbreak of hair defeat had struck again.

One of the most frustrating things about wearing straightened hair is trying to keep it that way — and live a normal, active life. We all know ladies who can't swim 'cause they refuse to ruin their hair.

You probably know some of the lifestyle rules for ladies who are serious to the point of murder about maintaining their 'do's.

RULE NO.1 Stay away from water or anything related to water. That means rain, light rain, snow, sleet, hail, fog, steam, bathrooms with hot showers going on, sprinklers and funky house parties. No boat rides.

RULE NO 2. No swimming allowed. Not unless you have a waterproof bathing cap and anyone who has tried one of these knows that a waterproof swim cap is an oxymoron. Trying to be cute and swimming with your head above the water usually doesn't work because the Peter Principle works against you and your hair *will* get wet. The exception to this rule is if you've scheduled a hair appointment after the swim. *Immediately* afterward.

RULE NO 3. No sweating or sweat inducing activities. That means serious jogging and aerobic exercise are out. Check out your popular jogging areas and notice how many ladies with serious do's are into aerobic *walking*. This also means no tennis dates that are immediately followed by lunch. How are you supposed to get your hair together?

RULE NO 4. Beware of the mighty hawk. No riding in convertibles or on motorcycles. If you go to fairs, carnivals and amusement parks, avoid the rides with the high hawk factor. You can't be cute with your hair standing up all over your head.

Of course, all these rules are suspended when you've gotten control of your hair and can enjoy life. Here are some things that I've found minimize hair disasters due to weather and lifestyle.

RAIN, FOG AND HUMIDITY

If your hair has been permanently straightened, you probably consider water or damp weather to be your enemy. Once you learn to stop overstraightening your hair, you will find that it has it's own natural body and come up with attractive ways to take advantage of its natural loops and waves when it responds to dampness and humidity. Curly hair loves moisture. The trick is to find a style that works with curls. If you go for a straight style that requires every hair to be in place, you'll be in for a big letdown.

I know that the hot, humid weather can be exhausting. There are times when it's impossible to do anything with your hair. But don't throw in the towel. Here's some ideas.

▶ **USE COMBS, BARRETTES, AND CLIPS FOR CONTROL.**

▶ **USE STYLES THAT ARE CONDUSIVE TO CURLY HAIR** — See "Wet Sets"

▶ **KEEP HAIR TRIMMED OR SHAPED IF YOU HAVE A PRECISION CUT.**

▶ **USE ALCOHOL-FREE GELS TO HOLD WAVES AND SEAL OUT MOISTURE.** Use it on the ends to help keep the curl bunches together. In general, the thinner, liquid gels are easier to work through your hair if it's really thick. The gelatinous gels are better for spot holding.

▶ **USE YOUR FINGERS TO SHAPE YOUR CURLS.** Combing separates the curl bunches and your hair will frizz.

▶ **REMEMBER THAT YOUR HAIR WILL TAKE LONGER TO DRY IN DAMP HEAT.** I experienced this myself in Puerto Vallarta, Mexico in 90 degree heat and 90 percent humidity. My scalp sweated profusely and I swam a lot so my hair always seemed damp. I wore a lot of twists, buns and straw hats during that vacation.

DAMP WEATHER HAIR STYLES

▶ **USE SILK SCARVES TO ENHANCE YOUR LOOK.** Get in the habit of carrying a scarf during bad weather months and you'll have a fighting chance if you're caught in bad weather.

▶ Scarves are a good enhancer for a bun or French twist when your hair line isn't as pretty as you'd like. Fold it into a wide headband and wear it around your hairline and put your hair up. Double wrap the scarf or twist and tuck in the ends so they don't dangle. Add a little make-up, some great earrings and you're ready to face the world!

▶ Rub some alcohol-free styling gel between your palms and slick your hair into a bun (if it's long) or a French twist (if it isn't very long but long enough to pin into one). Or part your hair in three or four sections and twist each section into a pretty roll. Pin up each roll.

▶ **FOR SHORT HAIR** Mix a quarter sized dab each of hair creme or pomade and liquid gel in the palm of your hand work it through your hair, encouraging little curls or waves

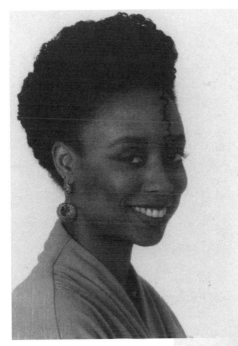

The corkscrew crimp upsweep or "Nefertiti" good for damp, humid or bad weather.

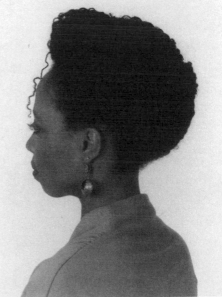

Back view of Nefertiti anchored with faux tortoiseshell hairpins.

The Movie Star Scarf Wrap

Good for convertibles, bad weather.

Add sunglasses for instant attitude

to form. Fold a scarf into a headband shape. Twist or wrap around your hair at the hairline. Arrange the little corkscrews into a halo.

▶ FOR LONGER HAIR Smooth gel through your hair and work it through the ends with your fingers so you'll have curly looking ends. Remember, don't comb it through or you'll end up with frizz. Take a scarf, fold it in a triangle and tie it on your head "Gypsy Style" with your curly ends framing the bottom. If you use a large enough scarf, you'll avoid the plantation look by twisting the ends, bringing them around the fabric on your forehead and tucking the ends around themselves.

HOT FUN IN THE SUMMERTIME

Because our African ancestry has blessed us with a skin protecting pigment called melanin, we tend to think we're immune to sun damage. We can tolerate more sun than lighter skinned races but if we lay out there long enough without protection, we'll be sunburned and peeling too. When it comes to our hair, it's pretty much the same story.

Our hair, unlike our skin, has no melanin to protect it. The most important thing to understand is that sunburned hair is like hair that has been burned with a blow dryer or curling iron. It will break off gradually and you'll be left searching for a style that will hide the damage.

You must also take special care of your hair when swimming in the ocean or pools. Salt water will dry and bleach your hair. Chlorinated pool water will bleach your hair and the chemicals used to fight algae can turn color treated hair into a green rainbow.

HOT WEATHER HAIR SURVIVAL

▶ USE SUN HATS if you know you're going to spend hours in the sun with little or no shade, say an outdoor concert, a day at the beach or hanging out in the park. It should be a hat with a brim. Don't forget to line it with a silk or satin scarf.

BONUS: People notice pretty ladies in hats and your make-up won't be baked into your skin after a day in the sun.

▶ **RINSE OUT SEA WATER AND CHLORINATED POOL WATER AFTER SWIMMING.** Shampoo with a build-up remover shampoo and follow with a moisturizing conditioner or a hair **equalizer**. Equalizers are conditioners designed to return the hair to its normal pH and close the cuticle. One that I've used with success is Aveda's Rosemary/Mint Equalizer for Hair and Scalp with Jojoba Oil.

▶ **SWIM CAPS.** Let's be real. The conventional ones leave you with drippy hair and a mean set of rings around your forehead that last for **hours.** Plus you feel like a dork when you and Grandma are the only eraserheads in the pool.

IF YOUR HAIR is permanently colored and chemically straightened, you should think seriously about wearing something because your hair is extremely vulnerable to damage. Try working conditioner through your hair before pinning it up. Then slip on one of those cool-looking racer swim caps like professional swimmers wear. You can find these in sporting goods stores. If you're swimming in a pool, wear some swim goggles on your forehead and you'll look cool.

▶ **NO SWIM CAP?** First, smooth a little conditioning hairdressing through your hair to minimize the effects of salt or chlorinated water. Then, if your hair is four inches or

HOT WEATHER
HAIR SURVIVAL

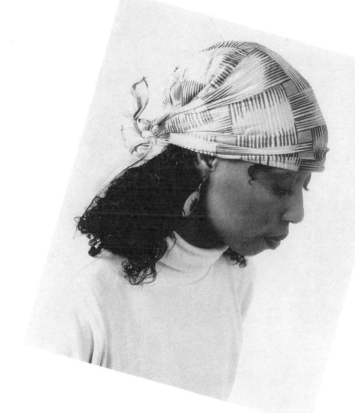

*This scarf wrap can go solo or
protect your hair from a wool
or straw`hat*

MORE HOT FUN

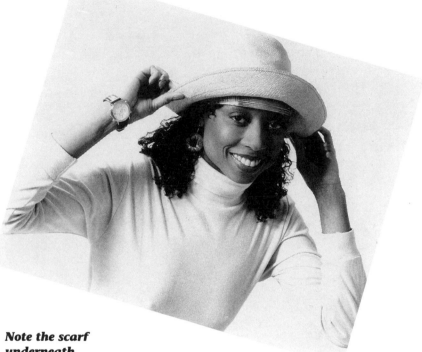

Note the scarf
underneath
the hat.

T H E B E A C H S E T

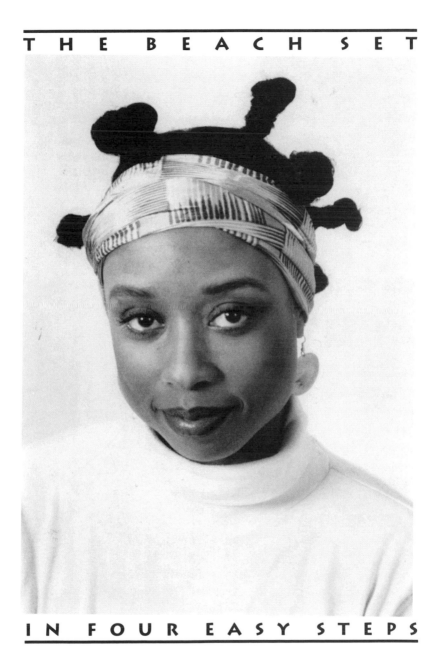

I N F O U R E A S Y S T E P S

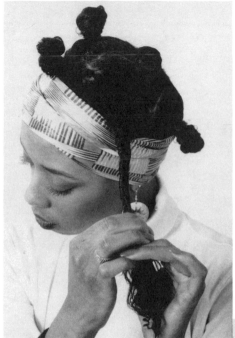

STEP 1

*Dampen section
of hair and twist
(The smaller the
section, the tighter
the curl.)*

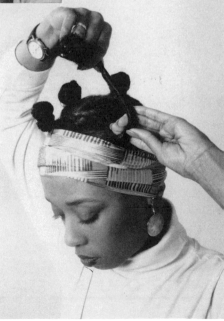

STEP 2

STEP 3

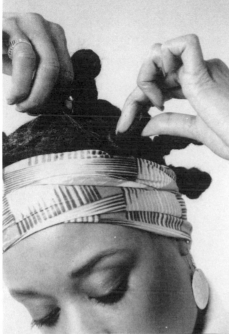

*Twist ends of hair
around the base
of the twist
Let dry and unfurl.
You'll have twisty,
curly waves.*

STEP 4

longer, do a couple of "milkmaid" twists on either side of your head or one French braid down the back. Be imaginative. What you are doing is protecting your hair from the corrosive action of the water and keeping it from tangling.

▶ **IF YOUR HAIR TURNS SLIGHTLY GREEN**, you can try a vinegar or lemon juice rinse. If it comes out closer to Joker Green, you'll have to consult a professional hairdresser.

COLD WEATHER AND THE MIGHTY HAWK

I've always been amazed to see how many ladies will go bareheaded in miserable weather, rather than wear something on their heads and "spoil" their hair style. The result is that the hair is damaged from exposure. Hair that is unprotected in extremely cold weather can snap and break and high winds will help dry it out and tangle it. If you've been smart enough to have a style that doesn't depend on rollers, blow dryers, curl activator or curling wands, you won't have a heart attack when the weather is bad and you've got to go out. You can wear proper head coverings and still look great when you remove them indoors.

COOL HAIR TIPS

▶ **WEAR PROTECTION** Wear hats lined with your reliable silk or satin scarf. The scarf prevents breakage caused by your hair rubbing against the rough fibers of the hat, even the soft wool knits.

▶ **PROTECT THE ENDS OF YOUR HAIR** by wearing twists or an upsweep. Remember, the ends are the oldest and most fragile part of your hair. Do some attractive twists that can hold up as a 'do throughout the day.

▶ **RIDING IN A CONVERTIBLE?** Try a ponytail or a French twist if you're zipping around town.

▶ **ZIPPING DOWN THE FREEWAY IN YOUR CON-VERTIBLE?** Be smart, don't be a human bug filter. Try a ba-a-a-d scarf, tied movie star style — tie it under your chin and tie the ends around your neck behind the scarf. Put on your shades and you'll be set.

In general, remember that simpler styles require less changes if you want to be active. Check out women with African hair in profesional sports — now there's inspiration for failsafe hair. The smarter ones have natural hair or a style that will stand up to heavy sweating and frequent shampooing. The others have the "rooster-in-flight" look or weaves.

Here's to Mo'Betta Hair!

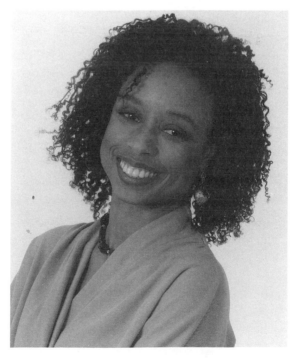

BIBLIOGRAPHY

Chase, Deborah — The New Medically Based No-Nonsense Beauty Book Henry Holt and Company 1989

Dalton, John W. — The Professional Cosmetologist. West Publishing Co. 1985

Gignac, Louis — Everything You Need To Know To Have Great Looking Hair. The Viking Press, 1981

Miliwcz, Felicia & Johnson, Lois Joy — The Beauty Editor's Workbook . Random House 1983

Morrison, Maggie — Glamour's Guide To Hair Conde Nast Publications 1986

Morrow, Willie — Curly Hair Morrow's Unlimited, Inc. 1973

Morrow, Willie — 400 Years Without A Comb Morrow's Unlimited, Inc 1973

Perelman, Suzanne & Lee, Mary — Natural Hair Care Comix & Stories. Straight Arrow Books 1973

Powlis, LaVerne — The Black Women's Beauty Book Doubleday 1979

Powlis, LaVerne — Beauty From The Inside Out Doubleday 1988

Sagay, Esi — African Hairstyles Heineman Educational Books, Inc 1983, 1985

Sims, Naomi — About Health and Beauty for the Black
    Woman, Doubleday 1976

Sims, Naomi — All About Hair Care For The Black
    Woman, Doubleday 1982

Vaughan-Richards, Ayo — Black & Beautiful
    Collins Publishing Co. 1986

PHOTOGRAPH
AND ILLUSTRATION CREDITS

Photographs

Pages 8 & 11—Courtesy of Lonnie and Dorothy Brittenum

Pages 22, 50, 58—Courtesy of Derek R. Bonner

Pages 28, 29, 47, 67, 73, 75, 76, 83, 84, 87, 88, 89, 90, 91, 93
and back cover photo—Auintard Henderson

Pages 65, 66, 68, 74—Victor Hall

Illustrations

Pages 16 & 17—Sergie Loobkoff

TEXTURIZING

So, what's the difference between texturizing hair and chemically straightening or relaxing hair?

With **chemical straightening**, a sodium hydroxide or thioglycolate based relaxer product is **smoothed** through tightly curled African hair until it has been **straightened.**

Chemically texturized hair results when a mild relaxer product is **combed** through the hair and left on a **few minutes** so it can **loosen** but not **straighten** tightly curled coils. Texturizing can be done using mild formulas of the traditional relaxer products currently available. The goal of texturizing is to achieve a **slightly loosened kink or curl that isn't far removed from your virgin hair texture.**

At this writing, there are home texturizer kits available over the counter, marketed primarily for men with short hair. However, unless you are extremely skilled, I suggest you let a professional perform any chemical work.

"U" PRONG ROLLERS

The "U" prong rollers are a product called "Perm for a Day."

They are manufactured by Uptown Products, Box 768, Fairfield, Iowa 52556, (515) 472-6875.

According to advertisements, they can also be purchased "at your favorite discount department store" and at Eckerd, Walgreens, CVS, Pharmhouse, Thrift Drug, Revco, Big Drugs, Thrifty, Peoples Drug, and Brooks.

NOTES